THE FIGHT OF OUR LIFE

A True Story of Crisis, Hope, and Love

Catherine Hawley

Toronto and New York

Copyright © 2014 by Catherine Hawley
All rights reserved. No part of this publication may be reproduced or transmitted in any form or by any means, electronic or mechanical, including photocopying, recording, or any information storage and retrieval system, without permission in writing from the publisher.

Published in 2014 by
BPS Books
Toronto and New York
www.bpsbooks.com
A division of Bastian Publishing Services Ltd.

ISBN 978-1-927483-96-1 (paperback)
ISBN 978-1-927483-98-5 (ePDF)
ISBN 978-1-927483-97-8 (ePUB)

Cataloguing-in-Publication Data available from Library and Archives Canada.

Cover: Gnibel
Text design: Tannice Goddard, www.bookstopress.com

Disclaimer: Some names and identifying details have been changed to protect the privacy of individuals in this book.

*To Bill,
my forever love*

CONTENTS

Preface xi

Acknowledgments xiii

Prologue 1

PART ONE
AND THEN THE DEMON STRUCK
1 "Something Is Wrong" 5
2 A Huge Assault 12
3 The Vigil 15
4 Unsuitable 20
5 Ups and Downs 25
6 Love at First Sight 29
7 A Godsend? 33
8 A Geriatric Warehouse 36
9 A Fine Mess 40

PART TWO
FROM FEAR TO ANGER

10	Seeking Balance	49
11	"The Right Thing"	51
12	Our Only Real Hope	57
13	Home Again	62
14	The New Bill	69
15	The Newest Assault	73
16	No Other Options	78
17	An Alien in a New Realm	83
18	Yes, Virginia…	92

PART THREE
A LITTLE LESS DRAMA, PLEASE

19	The Nag in His Life	99
20	D-Day	107
21	Unexplained Absences	111
22	"Things Just Happen"	117
23	A Private Cave	122
24	An Epiphany of Sorts	126
25	Definitely Not Homey	132
26	Attack and Retreat	141
27	Going AWOL	146
28	Teamwork	153
29	Tuesdays with Bill	160

PART FOUR
REHABILITATION, TOGETHER

30	Painting Lessons	167
31	A Real Shocker	174
32	Where the Rehab Is	178
33	Farther Down the Rabbit Hole	186
34	The Cavalry Almost Arrived	191
35	On the Road Again	197

36	At Cross-Purposes	202
37	Bureaucratic Compost	206
38	All I Needed to Know	211
39	Only Time Will Tell	214
40	At My Own Inquisition	219
41	"I Feel Like Crap"	224
42	"Might Not Be Going Home"	231
43	The Land of Denial	237
44	A Beautiful Life Together	241
45	The Underlying Cause?	243
	Appendix / Patient Beware	247

PREFACE

IN THE BEGINNING, WHEN my husband was undergoing brain surgery, I was the epitome of an "average" Canadian: I had no experience or education in the medical realm. I trusted, without question, that our health care system would always take care of him; would always do everything possible for his well being; would always keep him safe. But none of this was my experience.

Suddenly I was thrust into a new role: advocate for my husband as we encountered problems, crises, errors, and roadblocks. It is not my intention, in writing this book, to castigate the entire health care system but rather to point out some of the areas in which communication fails and mistakes are made (accidentally and frequently), all of which will require your own attention, caution, and persistence should you or a loved one face a medical crisis. Had I known more about the flaws in the system, the lessons I learned (so often too late) could have changed much of our story.

This book takes you, the reader, with us on our journey through the labyrinth of our health care system and brain injury, although many of the issues and problems we encountered relate to any complex illness or condition. Even to those that initially are simple and commonplace.

It is a cautionary tale, warning of things to be watchful for and vigilant about and ways to be proactive, and a love story, showing what commitment, dedication, persistence, tenacity, advocacy, and deep love can accomplish.

Our story became more complex than some, but it is by no means unique. Even in seemingly simple cases, things can go very wrong. What you don't know *can* hurt you.

ACKNOWLEDGMENTS

To EVERYONE WHO WAS part of our circle of support, both in doctors' offices, hospitals, and at home, thank you.

— My deepest gratitude to Dr. Michael Shirriff, Dr. Peter Ellis, Dr. Yolanda Madernos, and Dr. Allison Spiller: You are the very best of the best.
— My immense appreciation to our family and friends, especially to Judy and Andy, Brenda, Susan, Joyce and Earl, and Kevin: Your endless help, support, and encouragement helped make the doing possible.
— To the PSWs, nurses, managers, and other therapists who contributed so many positives: You know who you are, and all that you contributed to our journey, and I thank you sincerely.

And it took a circle of people to put this book in your hands. My thanks to:

— My writing buddy, Ray Herbert, whose never-ending encouragement and support and belief in this book helped me stay on the path.
— Sharon Stevens, Laurie Hill, and all the scribes in my writing groups and classes, for being such an encouraging, supportive audience from early days.
— Parise Herbert (Ray's wife), for so generously sharing all those hours and hours of Ray's time.
— Harry Goldhar, for teaching me how to sift the wheat from the chaff.
— Don Bastian, my editor and publisher, for his patience, guidance, and attention to detail to bring this project to life.

PROLOGUE

It was a virtual death sentence.

The resident at the hospital had just said, "We are recommending Bill be sent to a nursing home. He has some cognitive issues and is unlikely to benefit from rehabilitation."

Complications had set in ten days after *successful* brain surgery. Fewer than four weeks later, still unable to clearly define the cause, this medical team had reached its decision.

They were giving up on him.

My husband was fifty-six years old. It was my unshakeable belief that their decision was both wrong and premature. We had everything at stake. Suddenly I was fighting for his life. Our life.

How the hell did we get to this?

PART ONE

AND THEN THE DEMON STRUCK

I

"SOMETHING IS WRONG"

ONE EVENING LATE in the autumn of 2002, I was lounging, with my head on my husband's shoulder, when he whispered, "I need to tell you something, Hon."

The little hairs on my neck and arms stood to attention.

"Something is wrong," he said. "Something serious. I just know. I think I need to see the neurosurgeon."

Eyes squeezed tight, I nodded. He wrapped his arms around me. We hugged.

The CT scan and the subsequent MRI, both arranged by Dr. Michael Shirriff, our family doctor, confirmed Bill's suspicion and my fear. Just a few weeks past the tenth anniversary of his first surgery, he was diagnosed with a second brain tumour. Our doctor arranged for us to meet with a neurosurgeon at Kingston General Hospital, a university teaching hospital ninety-five kilometres to the east of our home in Trenton, Ontario.

On Friday, December 16, 2002, at six-thirty in the evening, we sat with that neurosurgeon, Dr. Peter Ellis, in a clinic room at Kingston General. Dr. Ellis appeared to have endless time and no thoughts other than of Bill.

Carefully, in plain language, he explained what he saw in the imaging. He pointed to a mass in the frontal lobe. He and Bill pointed to different squiggles in the CT scan images, each man asking direct questions, each giving direct answers. I stared at the squiggles in the carpet pattern, willing myself not to throw up.

The surgeon went over the pros and cons with us, and explained exactly what he would do during the surgery. Then he urged us to ask as many questions as we needed. He asked about our life, showing interest in Bill as a whole person, not just a specimen for surgery. We both felt complete confidence in him.

"I find it fascinating, Bill, that you've defied science for ten years," he said.

He was referring to Bill's medical history. His remark took me back to our previous experience.

On Thanksgiving weekend, 1992, after several days of memory loss and excruciating headaches, Bill was diagnosed with a brain tumour. Following emergency surgery that took place twelve hours later at Kingston General, the surgeon came to speak to us.

"Yes, it was quite a large and very aggressive-looking tumour," he said. "The surgery went very well, though."

But he gently indicated the prognosis was very poor.

Our experience in the hospital was very positive, with only a few minor glitches, but we were both relieved when the surgeon pronounced Bill fit for discharge. Recovery at home would be quieter and more peaceful. And the food would be better. Five days after major surgery, the patient was home, resting, recuperating, and downplaying the whole event.

Several weeks post-surgery, during an appointment with the oncologist at the Regional Cancer Clinic, attached to Kingston General, we were told "the pathology reports indicated the tumour was in fact "a very aggressive type of cancer. A type that no one survives."

The prognosis? Very, very poor. The impact of this information? Massive.

After letting us digest his words, the oncologist went on to say that, having conferred with his colleagues and having ruled out chemotherapy, he was willing to try the only available option: aggressive radiation. He warned us that, even with treatment, the prognosis was still very grim.

Bill underwent a lengthy course of daily radiation therapy. Five days a week for five weeks. By the halfway point, as we had been forewarned, fatigue set in, but he was fortunate to have no other significant side effects.

My husband had a remarkable outlook on his situation. He believed, heart and soul, the treatments would in fact work, and he was determined to live with a positive attitude, stay fit, mentally and physically, and be happy. His motto? "I am not going to live in fear for the rest of my life!"

Fully recovered, Bill went back to work five months after his surgery. I had come to understand that prognosis is not an exact science. All was well that ended well.

I DRAGGED MY mind back to our conversation with Dr. Ellis. He was speaking to both of us. He was very serious, but at the same time positive and encouraging.

"All that said, I'm confident I can 'de-bulk' this growth."

That was the information we had desperately wanted to hear. Had desperately hoped for. The only thing worse than learning you have a very serious condition is being told you have no options.

We left the doctor's clinic subdued but optimistic. We would get through this, just like the last time. Of course we would.

BILL'S SURGERY DATE, January 5, 2003, rolled in on us very quickly. We arrived at the hospital at six o'clock in the morning, as requested.

An hour and a half passed before a resident came out to tell us the surgery had been postponed. There had been had an overnight emergency — a huge car crash with many injured — and no operating rooms were available.

We endured three more postponements over the next fifteen days. Twice we were already inside the hospital. The first three times we remained calm, acknowledging that emergencies come up, that there are only so many operating rooms and only so many surgeons. Postponement number four sent me into total fear. Imagining the tumour growing faster and faster, I phoned our Member of Parliament. He offered to make inquiries. Two days later, January 30, at six-thirty in the morning, my husband was finally in surgery. The politician's intervention? The squeaky wheel? Probably both.

It was a very long day. Our closest friends, Joyce and Earl, who also lived in Trenton, and Bill's sister Judy, who flew in from her home in Berwick, Nova Scotia, seventeen hundred kilometres away, took turns keeping me company. Sitting, standing, pacing, and praying in the secluded waiting room, I was afraid to leave for more than a couple of minutes. Just in case. Hours later, when I saw Dr. Ellis coming down the hall, my heart started racing and my stomach lurched. I was petrified he was going to say something had gone horribly wrong during the operation.

Instead, he announced, grinning ever so slightly, "The surgery went very well. No neurological damage. Bill will be in the neuro critical care unit shortly, just for observation. Now we just wait to see how things go."

All I could do was bear-hug him, I was so relieved.

I expected the next few days to be relatively uneventful: a gradual move back to normal for my husband now that the tumour had been annihilated. Just like the first time.

Later that evening Bill was moved from the neuro critical care unit to a regular room on the neurology floor. On one level, I took it as a sign he was stable and out of danger. On a second level, though,

I was afraid of leaving the neuro critical care cocoon, where a nurse would watch him constantly. I stayed so he wouldn't be alone whenever he woke up.

Just before midnight, I was dozing, my head resting on Bill's arm, when I felt a vibration, which grew stronger by the second. Suddenly Bill's whole body erupted into motion, twisting and writhing. His face contorted. His eyes rolled about in their sockets. Then suddenly they went vacant. Dead-looking.

I flew into the hall, shouting for help. Nurses came running. In a few minutes they assured me it was *just* a grand mal seizure. When I realized they were going to leave him unattended I expressed my serious concerns.

The resident sounded patronizing. "Seizures like this aren't unusual after brain surgery."

"What if it happens again? What if it's worse? What if he chokes? If you don't know he's having seizures, how will you know to adjust his anti-seizure medication? He shouldn't be alone."

"You should go home and rest, Mrs. MacLeod. Otherwise you won't be able to help him later."

I had kept my maiden name when I married Bill, but had decided to answer to Mrs. MacLeod in the hospital. Things were getting complicated enough without confusing the staff with names.

"I would go home if I felt some degree of confidence that you'll keep him alive until morning," I said. "That someone will know if he's not okay. You do realize that he had a seizure disorder before the surgery, don't you?"

I wasn't usually rude or demanding or hysterical, but I was shocked by what seemed to be the callous indifference of the resident and the nurses toward both Bill and me. For medical people it was just business as usual, but for me it was very frightening. I thought Bill should be moved back to the neuro critical care unit where he would be watched constantly.

The little I did know was that the anti-seizure drug would need adjusting. I was paralyzed by the fear of those horrific seizures striking again, and I wasn't going to risk his being alone if they did. I stayed all night, holding his hands, hoping I would be able to help him, comfort him, if it happened.

As bad luck would have it, it did: two times. The motion pictures seared themselves into my mind. No one on staff would have known or helped him if I hadn't been there. The first seed of fear was planted. I had never realized the importance of having someone with you as much as possible while in a hospital.

THE NEXT MORNING, January 31, Bill pushed the help button for assistance getting to the bathroom, as he'd been told to do. He pushed it again five minutes later. And five minutes later again. No one answered the bell. Determined not to use a bedpan, and before I could get over to help him, he swung his legs over the side of the bed. As he stood up, he lost his balance and fell, tumbling through the curtain onto the patient in the next bed and then onto the floor. Suddenly three nurses were at hand, available to get him back into bed. Where had they been earlier?

My husband had been put in jeopardy twice already, and it was only day two.

I tried to assist however I could, fetching things, fluffing pillows, helping Bill wash his face and eat, but I definitely was not equipped to take on nursing work. And it seemed to me that many nurses routinely ignored call bells and lights. Often I'd walk out into the hallway and see several staff gathered at the nursing station chatting or doing paperwork, not getting up to provide help when patients were in need. I started going out to the nursing station whenever Bill's call bell wasn't answered within ten minutes. I planted myself in front of the desk and waited until someone would follow me to his room.

Thankfully, since there were no imminent issues left to deal with, Bill was discharged by the surgeon less than a week later, on February 4. While the staff had found Bill charming and sweet, I am certain they were grateful to see the last of me, the newly paranoid wife.

And so Bill came home with me, walking, talking, and teasing me about having to live off my cooking for a while. We expected life to get back to normal relatively soon. Just like the first time.

2

A HUGE ASSAULT

And then the demon struck.

When I woke up on February 13, Bill was breathing but appeared to be unconscious. I phoned Dr. Shirriff, who urged me to get Bill to the local hospital, which was just five minutes from our home. He would call the neurosurgeon. In less than an hour we were in an ambulance, on our way back to Kingston General.

The ER staff there examined, prodded, and consulted, comparing theories and solutions. They did a CT scan and a multitude of other tests but found no definite explanation. Dr. Ellis spoke with me at Bill's bedside.

"Bill's brain has endured a huge assault through surgery," he said. "It might simply be overwhelmed and shutting down to allow further healing. It's not all that uncommon. Try not to worry. We'll keep a close eye on him."

I found comfort in his words and knew Bill was in the best possible hands.

Within a few days, my husband was alert again, walking, talking, eating, and anxious to be on his way home, where we returned on February 17.

One week later, though, the crisis reoccurred. The ER staff in our local hospital contacted the neurosurgery staff at Kingston General and explained Bill's condition. Kingston General agreed a neurosurgery assessment was vital, but they were very clear they would not be able to keep him in their hospital this time: no beds were available that day.

The residents and neurosurgeon examined Bill, did another CT scan, and ran more tests. Dr. Ellis thought it likely Bill had experienced a low-grade seizure in his sleep. I asked about the steroid medication Bill was taking. He listened carefully as I explained Bill's hyper-sensitivity to drugs in the past and said, "Yes, that could be a connection." After he contacted the ER doctor in Trenton and discussed the case, we were ferried back to that hospital. We never heard from or saw that ER doctor again.

Once back in our local hospital, I soon discovered that, while they did in fact have beds, they did not have any doctors or nurses with expertise in brain surgery. Bill remained virtually comatose in their special care unit for five days. He was on an IV, but the doctors appeared to be doing nothing else.

Being a "buffet Catholic" — that is, I pick and choose what I like — I was surprised to find myself offering up anything and everything to God if he would help us. I sat by Bill's bed, holding his hands to keep our connection strong, recalling special moments, thinking about our future, and praying.

Early on the fourth morning, February 22, I lay in wait to speak to the attending doctor. When I asked what was happening, desperate for any information, he said, "I should think that is fairly obvious."

It certainly wasn't obvious to me. He became Dr. ASOB (arrogant son of a bitch) in my mind.

Even our family doctor, who had practicing privileges at this hospital, was unable to intervene. He wasn't the attending physician and therefore couldn't tell these specialists what to do. The next day the nurse who had been with Bill for several days pleaded with them at least to let her call the neurosurgeon for a second opinion. They finally relented.

In two hours we were in an ambulance en route to Kingston General, again.

I realized then I should have raised holy hell to have him remain in care there in the first place. A bed in a hallway with the right specialists on staff would have been safer than a private room in a place where they knew very little about Bill's kind of issues.

Once Bill was checked in, a careful, thorough young resident examined him. I watched her go back to the x-ray box, time after time, and peer at his chest x-ray. Something wasn't right. She discovered a tiny speck. It was, in fact, a blood clot in his lung.

"These are usually only found post-mortem," she told me.

"Thank you, Doctor, for listening to your instincts, and for your persistence," I replied, knowing the gods were taking this seriously.

Was this the root problem? Could this be the cause of these near comas? The doctors put Bill on blood thinners, inserted an indwelling catheter, and continued to monitor him.

Dr. Ellis weighed in on the most likely cause of Bill's bouts of unresponsiveness.

"Prolonged low-grade seizures. Possibly could be related to the clot. We just have to keep monitoring him now and see what's up."

The next morning, February 24, I was told that, with tumour and surgery-related complications ruled out, Bill wouldn't be under the neurosurgeon's care any more. He was being passed over to the neurology department staff.

3

THE VIGIL

THE NEUROLOGY TEAM, INCLUDING a troop of med students, breezed through early most mornings, but they had very little information to share with me.

"The blood thinner is doing its job, but we have no real plan yet," was a typical comment.

Sitting in the neuro critical care unit again, I was afraid of leaving Bill's side. Holding his hand was the only thing that seemed real. Tubes and monitors surrounded us. Every beep and every change in the numbers produced a jab of fear in me, even though I had no idea what they meant. After three days he was still not responding, except to touch. And I wondered if I was just imagining *that* response. Was it wishful thinking? I tried to comprehend the difference between a coma and an unresponsive state. Looked like a coma to me.

The unit itself had five or six beds, two enclosed by glass partitions.

Bill had been in one of those after his first surgery.

Megan and Sandra, two of the nurses caring for him now, were indirectly caring for me, too. They were so gentle with him, constantly checking all his equipment and monitors. They brought me warm blankets, dispensed a pat on the shoulder, and offered explanations every time they did something to or for Bill. The nurses' attention to detail was remarkable; it helped that, in this unit, they usually had only two patients each. A phone rang constantly at the desk. People who couldn't be with their loved one could get updates twenty-four hours a day.

I knew how fortunate I was to be able to sit here and touch Bill and watch. The big windows showed if it was day or night. A large clock let me watch the minutes and hours and days trail by.

Joyce and Earl were with us, as well as Bill's sister Judy, who had flown back for the second time from Nova Scotia as soon she heard about this serious complication. All three stayed close, right outside the unit door. They were in fear and prayer mode, too. Joyce and Judy made phone calls, updating both families. I couldn't talk to anyone yet, couldn't say, out loud, that we still didn't know what was wrong. They sat with Bill when I went out to fortify myself with coffee and a cigarette. This was very painful for them, too. They talked to Bill as if he were wide awake, keeping him up to speed on the world at large.

I knew my sister, Brenda, and sister-in-law, Brenda Lee, were taking care of our non-hospital needs by looking after Jessie, our puppy, and rescheduling my appointments with clients. I had owned my own salon in Toronto for more than fifteen years, but when we decided to move to Trenton I opted to rent space in another salon in Toronto, and make the one-and-a-half-hour commute. Hard as it was to concentrate on anything other than Bill, practical things still needed to be done.

Our vigil continued. We waited and waited and waited. For several days there was little or no change. No responses. No improvement. I was full of fear, not knowing when, if ever, he was going to come around again.

And so I prayed. "Please, please, God, don't take him from me. I can't believe you would be so cruel. Bill hasn't lived enough yet, and I am way too young to be a widow, damn it!"

People in unresponsive states are believed to be aware, at some level, of what is going on, so I talked to him constantly. I knew he was listening. I struggled to sound calm and casual because I wanted him to know, to believe, he would be okay. I didn't want him to be scared.

"Jessie Puppy has been chasing squirrels and playing a real game with them. She also burrowed in the snow and made herself a little cave. Not easy to find your white dog in a white snow cave, Hon. You have a ton of cards to read when you wake up. I'm thinking of getting my hair cut short, the way you like it."

As I chattered on and on, I wondered if he was lying there thinking, "For God's sake, Cath, please shut up for a while!"

Occasionally an arm or leg moved, and my heart skipped a beat. I was certain he was finally waking up. No, just a twitch. I learned about voluntary and involuntary movements. The critical care unit became my universe. Time seemed suspended as we waited, and waited, and waited.

Then suddenly I felt, more than saw, something change. His eyelids fluttered, one at a time, very, very slowly. Just a flicker. Then nothing. Time stopped. I went back into my prayers, bargaining with God.

And then, there it was again! As minutes dragged by, stubbornly, slowly, both beautiful hazel eyes gradually opened. Finally, a week after he became unresponsive, he was waking up. Relief washed over me like a tsunami.

My husband was back.

But his expression baffled me. Bill didn't seem to grasp who I was or what he was looking at. I gathered him into our usual bear hug and felt him relax into me. It was, as always, a perfect fit. He was coming back. At that moment I knew it for sure. "Thank you, God," I whispered.

After five days of improvement, Bill was moved out of the neuro critical care unit into a regular room down the hall. I knew this meant he was more stable, but now I was even more afraid of his being alone. Afraid bad things would happen and no one would know. For a week I stayed in his room night and day, worried no one would notice any changes in him, good or bad.

When he was more wakeful and his brain more rested, he would be his old self, I thought. I relied on the "smooch test" to see how he was doing. Each time I left the room and came back, I asked for my kiss. The degree of "pucker up" told me how he was, cognitively, at that very moment. This was a true assessment. I knew him better than the staff — very differently from them, too.

I learned quickly that in a teaching hospital there is a rotation of doctors, residents, and interns. Each new group brings new issues, new opinions, and new theories. It worried me that it seemed to be the residents who were forming the opinions and plans and passing them on to the specialist, not the other way around.

Every two days brought a rotation of new nurses, as well, which made it difficult for any of them to notice changes, good or bad, from day to day.

I asked one of them, "How could anyone, nurse or doctor, even begin to know the status and progress of any patient in two days, especially someone unable to speak for himself?"

"Therein lies part of the problem," she replied grimly.

Midway through the second or third week after Bill was readmitted, and with significant weight loss obvious, the doctors inserted a gastric tube through Bill's nose into his stomach. It was horribly invasive, but in his semi-conscious state, it was the only way to get nutrition into his body. I wished they had done it sooner. Bill started to improve, albeit in tiny increments. But still no one gave me a conclusive explanation for the complications or offered any ideas about what they anticipated.

I was just stumbling along waiting for him to recover.

Each doctor's visit started with, "Hi, Mr. MacLeod. Do you know where you are? Do you know what day it is? Do you know why you are here?"

My mind, but not my voice, answered for him, "Of course Mr. MacLeod doesn't know where the hell he is. He went to sleep in his own bed, in his own home, and woke up somewhere different surrounded by strangers!"

4

UNSUITABLE

Two books came into my life when I desperately needed them: *Where Is the Mango Princess? A Journey Back from Brain Injury* by Cathy Crimmins and *On Family, Hockey and Healing* by Walter Gretzky. As I read and connected with much of each person's experience, I realized my husband's circumstances and condition would be more aptly described as "brain injury" now, which changed how I looked at his care.

Where is the Mango Princess? recounts the story of an American man who'd sustained a head injury in a boating accident while on vacation in Canada. He'd been treated in this very hospital, by the same surgeon. With that book, I started the process of learning about brain injury. Details on the ways it could manifest itself and the process of rehabilitation were invaluable. I was comforted by the remarks of the author, the man's wife, about Kingston General. She dreaded going home to the United States because, in

Canada, her husband would immediately go into brain injury rehab. I was relieved to know we were in such good hands, with such a great system. Grateful to be Canadian.

Not knowing she was very misinformed about accessibility to rehab in Canada, I took encouragement from her story. I started reading everything I could about brain tumours, brain injury, medications, and anything else I thought pertinent. I realized it was important for me to know and understand as much as possible about Bill's condition.

The other book was Walter Gretzky's story about his recovery after his stroke, which is another form of brain injury. It offered great insight into the practical aspects of recovery. The rehabilitation he received was the difference between a life of quality and one of very limited quality, possibly even death. Mr. Gretzky detailed the need for structure, consistency, repetition, and positive reinforcement, including the need to control stimulation: not too much, not too little. He credited the positive attitude of everyone around him for his recovery.

What I didn't learn, though, was what to do if your son *isn't* Wayne Gretzky.

AS THE LONG, fearful days rolled by, I watched, listened, and learned things I had never wanted to know. I realized Bill's short-term memory was impaired, but not his long-term. When I read cards from friends and family, he knew who each person was. Keeping him oriented became my mission. Tips from my reading started to come in handy. I bought a dry-erase whiteboard and wrote the day and date on it. I left notes reminding him where I was and when I would be back. If a test was scheduled, I wrote it on the board. I wrote the hospital name and his room number at the top so he could read it and hopefully remember where he was. I also brought in his favourite music and photos. Reminders of home.

By week three he was consistently remembering where he was. Tears ran down my face the morning he said, "These doctors have crappy memories. They keep asking me the same questions every day."

After three weeks in bed, his balance was askew. His muscles were weakening. The physiotherapist worked with him on many days but had time only for very short sessions. I feared this was going to be far too little. In week three he was still able to stand, briefly, holding onto the hands of the neurologist, but I feared that, without a lot more help, he would continue to lose more strength and focus.

One afternoon, standing in the doorway to Bill's room, while orienting a new resident about Bill and his chart, Dr. Lind, the senior neurology resident, said, too loudly, "Oh, that's Mr. MacLeod. His brain is fried."

I flew into the hallway, screaming like a shrew.

"Who the hell do you think you are? Have you never studied any psychology? Bill isn't deaf. He and all these other patients hear your thoughtless, offhand, negative comments. So much for encouraging people to recover!"

I worried about the people on this floor who didn't have someone around all the time to help them reconnect and to augment their care. Without a family member or friend to advocate for them, especially where complicated or cognitive issues were apparent, was their care as comprehensive as it should have been?

When I started asking the staff about rehabilitation programs, I got mixed messages. I had an uneasy feeling this medical team and I were not on the same page. Almost daily I badgered the neurology team to have Bill assessed for a program. They finally agreed.

I was frustrated and disappointed to learn the physiatrist from the rehab centre did assessments only on Thursdays. It was already evident to me, and to many of the staff, that Bill was far more responsive when I was with him. At this point in Bill's medical travails I had just gone back to work, but only two days a week, on Thursdays and Fridays. I felt I really couldn't take more time off to be present for the appointment but wished fervently that I could.

In the end I was told that Bill fell far short of their criteria for brain injury rehab and was deemed unsuitable for the program.

I became acutely aware of how hospital care had changed over the years since our initial experience ten years prior. That visit, by comparison, was a slam-dunk. Now I was never clear about who was overseeing Bill's progress, or who was making the important recommendations and decisions. It seemed, from my vantage point, that the residents were forming their opinions and the specialists were accepting them as "most probable."

As soon as the staff could transfer Bill into a wheelchair, I started taking him to the lounge where there were huge windows overlooking the waterfront. Away from his hospital room he made slow and steady but significant progress with eating and talking. We read short items in the newspapers together and watched news on TV. We chatted about family and Jessie, and about how, very soon, we would be back in our home together. My husband was coming back, slowly but surely.

My unexpected, and previously unwanted, medical education was well underway. The patient care assistants taught me how to operate the mechanical lift, used with patients who couldn't get from bed to chair on their own. I learned about skin care problems, too. They even showed me how to make the bed with Bill in it. And some of the nurses shared their knowledge about seizures and urinary tract infections. On the one hand, I was a reluctant learner, but on the other, I knew this learning process was necessary.

Even my language had shifted. I became fluent in institutional vernacular. I learned about the negative effects on Bill of dehydration and low sodium levels, what high and low potassium levels cause, triggers for seizures, and the difference between sensitivities and allergies. And that the effects of these issues on each patient are individual and can be extremely important. Life and death important.

Medically, Bill was stabilizing, although new issues came and went. Daily, I told the "new" nurses about the gains he *was* making, naturally focusing on the positive aspects. I brought pictures of us taken a week after his surgery, to help them see him as a whole person, not just a medical complication or chart. I needed them to understand he was a determined and optimistic man, one who, with help, could overcome much.

Often I received a tolerant, patronizing gaze for my troubles — what I soon realized was the wife-in-denial look.

Late at night I researched information on drugs. Although Dr. Ellis and I had previously talked about Bill's hypersensitivity to drugs, the neurology team didn't seem to consider it a factor. I asked residents and nurses alike if the Decadron could be affecting him negatively

"Did you know this drug can cause hyper-somnolence [extensive periods of deep sleep], confusion, muscle weakness? Could this be part of the problem?"

My questions were brushed off by all, but the issue nagged at me. Bill had eight out of ten of the most common side effects. Why wouldn't anyone listen? At least consider my concern? At least look into it?

5

UPS AND DOWNS

Those four weeks since Bill was readmitted into the neuro critical care unit and turned over to the neurology department were a series of ups and downs. He slipped into three separate episodes of decreased level of consciousness.

The first was traced to an infection. He was given antibiotics and rebounded within a few days. I wondered if the infection stemmed from the catheter that had been inserted.

The second was traced to toxicity of Dilantin, his anti-seizure medication.

"How do medication levels get too high, here in a hospital where they're being monitored?" I thought.

The drug was withheld until his levels adjusted.

In the third episode, the cause was labelled "metabolic," a word way beyond my scope of understanding.

AND THEN, JUST a month after Bill had been readmitted to this hospital and put in the hands of the neurology department, I was asked to attend a "family meeting." This was to discuss the details of when Bill would be discharged from the hospital. I anticipated that Bill's progress would continue to be steady, if considerably slower than ideal. I thought they would recommend increased therapy to get him up and out, and tell me what else we could do to be homeward bound.

I was very, very wrong.

"Mrs. MacLeod, the team had a patient care discharge planning meeting yesterday, and we are recommending Bill be sent to a nursing home," said Dr. Lind, speaking for the medical team that had been caring for Bill. "He has some cognitive issues and is unlikely to benefit from rehabilitation. We believe Bill's circumstances require institutional care. We don't think he is safe to return home."

I realized that Dr. Lind, the resident who had said Bill's brain was "fried," had been a principal in assessing Bill's prognosis and deciding his future. Clearly he had formed his opinion a long time ago. Around the table in the conference room with Dr. Lind were the physio and occupational therapists, the nurse manager, the liaison from Community Care Access Centre, the social worker, and me, "the wife."

"Pardon me?" I asked.

"You would never be able to manage this much care at home, and…"

I interrupted whatever was coming next.

"But he's getting better," I said. "He's much more alert, he's talking more, and he's eating much better. Even the nurses see a big difference. He doesn't need to be a hundred per cent to go home. We will do whatever we have to do to keep him improving. We need help, not an institution. Please, it's only been a few weeks. You can't give up on him this soon."

No one said anything, so I continued: "My husband is fifty-six years old. There is not a chance in hell I am going to let you dump him into an institution! Surely you can't decide something this life shattering in a matter of weeks? You don't know anything about Bill's determination, or about us, or about what we're willing to do to get back home together. There has to be a way."

By now I was begging.

"We will do whatever it takes for him to progress," I said, "but I will not let you do this. Please help us."

"Catherine, we all shared our opinions," the social worker said. "This is the best thing for Bill."

Everyone nodded their agreement.

Dr. Lind reiterated their position. "We don't think Bill would be safe anywhere else, and he will require far too much care to go home. I'm sorry. "

He stood, picked up his notes, and left.

For another fifteen minutes the rest of my husband's medical team, who now felt more like the enemy, talked about my going to see a few nursing homes nearer to where we lived. They gave me their overview of what the care would be, and how it might be different from one institution to another. Someone explained how the fees for nursing home care were structured, and what was covered by the health care system and what was not. They shared their thoughts and recommendations, implying that they knew much more than I did about what was best for my husband. Each one ended by saying that putting my husband in an institution would be much easier for me.

Apparently I hadn't articulated that easy wasn't one of my priorities. Easy was the last thing on my mind when faced with this ultimatum. I couldn't believe they were giving up without giving him a fair time margin for further recovery, without considering other options for us. I didn't say any more, because I was afraid I would lose control completely and because I already understood there was no point.

The irony of the name of this meeting struck me. How could they have a family planning meeting that did not include my opinion? Apparently I was supposed to simply accept their proclamation.

It was now late March. This medical team had cared for Bill for a month. They were still unable to clearly define the cause of his condition, but they had reached a decision. They were giving up on him.

I realized I was now fighting for his life, for our life, for our future. I didn't realize it would be the fight of our life.

IN THE WASHROOM, as I washed away the tearstains and put on fresh lipstick, I rehearsed my best, most positive smile. Back in Bill's room we resumed our activities. We talked, and I read "get well" cards. We listened to his favourite music. I helped him with his meal. He was managing his food much better now. How could they not see how much he had improved over a few weeks?

After the evening nurse had been in and Bill was settled for the night, I took my leave. I drove the hour back to Trenton, forcing my mind to focus on the country music station's repertoire, hoping to clear my head and my heart of the fear, anger, and frustration that were settling on me like a dark, ugly shroud.

6

LOVE AT FIRST SIGHT

ONCE INSIDE THE WALLS of our home, though, the impact of the meeting took over. I hurled my purse across the room, kicked my shoes against the wall with a vengeance, and slumped onto the couch. Hoover Dam was crumbling.

I closed my eyes, and in the time between two heartbeats, my memory whisked me back to the very beginning of our life together and all that was at stake now.

It was Thanksgiving 1984. I'd flown from my home in Toronto to Nova Scotia, to stay at my parents' home in Ingonish, Cape Breton. My father was critically ill in the tiny hospital there. He and my mother had recently moved back to Ingonish, his hometown, when he retired from the police force in Toronto.

Of all things, my mother was having company. Plans made previously, she insisted. Was she matchmaking? Surely not.

There he was, by the fireplace in my parents' living room. Tall, slim, and standing almost at attention, he was an extremely attractive man. As we were introduced, I took in details: dark, thick hair with streaks of silver at the temples, impeccable grooming, a perfectly trimmed moustache, and a big, bright, inviting smile. I looked into the hazel eyes. They were staring directly back into mine. Was that a twinkle? Or an appraisal?

Conversation flowed easily, and I was infatuated by the time dinner was on the table. By dessert, my mother was all but invisible.

We never had a moment of awkward silence. There was so much to talk about. Bill had grown up in Cape Breton, just like my dad. He had left home to join the military, just like my dad. Returning to his home town of Ingonish after many years of service in the Air Force, he had set to work restoring his childhood home, expecting to remain there. We shared stories about our families, and talked about work, friends, philosophies, and life. It felt as if we had known each other forever.

"So, is there a significant man in Toronto?" Bill asked.

"No. And, for the record, I am not even remotely in the market for a boyfriend, live-in, or husband. It's only my mother who wants to see me married off. I like being on my own. I don't compromise easily, and I definitely don't share very well: space or toothpaste."

"Whoa," he said, chuckling. He put his hands out in front of his body as if to fend off my tirade.

Our first encounter extended into the dawn. We watched the sun come up over the deep blue Atlantic. I loved his humour. Dry, subtle. He was well read, well spoken, well informed. That we both found the ocean soothing and calming and mysterious was intriguing. By breakfast I understood the phrase "love at first sight."

For several months we met every weekend. I flew to Halifax to visit my father, who had been moved to a hospital there, while Bill drove the four-hour trip from his home. Those weekends were a roller coaster of emotions. We had a whirlwind affair, falling *in love and in lust in record time. Ours was never a smouldering passion. More like spontaneous combustion.*

Our long-distance romance was the good part of our early story. Sadly, my father did not recover. When he died it was, without question, the most crushing event of my life. He had been a major influence in my life. To him, I was always the perfect, if sometimes wayward and free-spirited, daughter. It seemed implausible to me that life would in fact go on.

Throughout this very personal crisis, Bill simply wrapped his arms around me, a lifeline for me in my grief. How strange to have the very worst experience of your life intertwined with the very best experience of your life. We continued to unearth more and more about each other. We rang up enormous phone bills during our nightly talks, but a romance like this was priceless. We were incredibly at ease, always able to share everything about ourselves with complete honesty. Unconditional love is very, very rare.

Bill's two-week visit with me in Toronto that Christmas in 1984 was a wonderful diversion. We shared and laughed and cried. But mostly laughed. He was taking care of me, and I revelled in the warmth of his attention. I'd never known such an orderly, disciplined person. It was unfathomable to me that someone would hang their shirts, pants, and ties in a colour sequence. I, in contrast, could rarely find two shoes that matched without a hunt. We loved and laughed and acted like love-struck teenagers much of the time.

Too quickly, it was time for Bill to return home to his real life. The night before his flight he offered an ultimatum.

"Will we have a life together or not? I am not cut out for long-distance love, and I am not willing to settle for it. This has to be all or nothing."

Clearly, it was my decision to make. Equally clearly, he wasn't going to ask a second time. Already deeply in love, I voted to jump in with abandon.

This was the man I wanted to share every second of the rest of my life with. That he loved me so completely and thoroughly, in spite of my quirks, astonished and delighted me. We both recognized this as a once-in-a-lifetime love.

Leaving his maritime life behind, Bill moved to Toronto, and within the year, we were married. Together we planned and built a new home in the country near Uxbridge, a small town about forty kilometres northeast of Toronto, where the peace and quiet and privacy suited us well. We worked well and comfortably together, tackling almost everything hand-in-hand. We had the space and privacy to enjoy our collection of dogs and the outdoor life we both loved.

Several years later, when an appealing opportunity to rejoin his former military life came up — a position in the Air Force Reserves — we made the move to Trenton, a military town, still within commuting distance of my business.

Pictures flashed through my mind of the years of quiet dinners, vacations, day trips, snowshoeing, the pets we loved, and the crazy fun and laughter we shared every day. Our life had been very, very good.

Coming to with a start, tears cascaded down my face. My heart ached for the life we had shared until so recently.

7

A GODSEND?

THE NEXT DAY THE social worker approached me.

"Great news, Catherine! We can get Bill into the Complex Continuing Care unit in Trenton Hospital. They have physio and occupational therapy and he'll be close to home. All the help he needs and right in your local hospital."

For a moment I was suspicious of this new plan, in that split second when, after asking if I could go to see their set-up, she said, "Well, no, you won't be able to go to see it first, but there's no need." But, desperate to keep them from declaring Bill disposable, I didn't want to question anything that sounded hopeful. Optimism and encouragement somehow rose from the ashes.

Two days later, on March 26, severe acute respiratory syndrome (SARS) was declared a provincial emergency and a hold was put on all hospital transfers. No patients could be moved between hospitals. For us it was a blessing. The ban on patient transfers lasted four weeks, during which time Bill made significant gains.

One day I snuck a peek at his chart. There were notations by residents that reported, "Patient says he feels well today, and he looks it." "Very alert, eating well, remembering staff names, very well oriented."

I thought, "Yes, now they're seeing his progress, too. Thank God."

I trusted that, based on their own notes, the team would reconsider their decision and adjust their plan and prognosis of "not likely to benefit from rehabilitation." But no.

At the end of April, Bill, accompanied by his friend Earl, went by stretcher to the Regional Cancer Clinic next to KGH for his standard three-month follow-up appointment. Two days later, the day Bill was being transferred to Trenton Hospital, his oncologist from that clinic, Dr. Yolanda Madernos, surprised us by checking on him in his room at KGH.

"I wanted to meet you personally, Mrs. MacLeod, and go over things with you and Bill together. Right now there is absolutely no need for chemotherapy. The most recent imaging shows no evidence of residual malignant disease." Turing to me she said, "But even if he had needed it, I couldn't even consider giving it in his present condition."

Dr. Madernos was concerned about Bill's de-conditioned state. She advised us to focus on getting him built up physically to be a good candidate for chemo if or when it became necessary.

I asked her why Dr. Ellis had been so keen for Bill to have what they said was a newer, better type of chemotherapy.

"I think Dr. Ellis did an even better job than he realizes," she said.

Leaving Bill's room, she stopped to speak to the resident who would be writing the discharge papers. I overheard her repeat exactly what she had just shared with us. The young woman, whose English, I had noticed, was rather limited, nodded and made a note without asking any questions.

It was now the beginning of May. We had been at Kingston

General for two months. Despite all the issues that had arisen, I was grateful for our health system and the people who struggled to make it work well, and I was doing my best to see the unit he was being transferred to in Trenton as a godsend.

The paramedics transferred Bill to a gurney and collected the discharge paperwork from the nurses' station. Bill waved goodbye, all smiles, and I shed a few tears of gratitude. But several things disturbed me: The team had made the decision to send Bill to a nursing home four weeks earlier, as far as I could tell without input from the oncologist or the neurosurgeon. He was still on a lot of different drugs, including the steroid I had practically stopped asking about. I felt inept for not knowing more and understanding better.

8

A GERIATRIC WAREHOUSE

As we exited the elevator to the Complex Continuing Care unit at Trenton Hospital with the paramedics, I couldn't hold back a gasp. My brain tried desperately not to process what my eyes were seeing: that dreadful drab grey-green of hospitals long ago. A long, dim, narrow hallway stretched ahead of us, full of various carts and equipment and a number of ancient bodies in wheelchairs, some of them moaning, others wailing.

This was to be Bill's new home? "Oh my God, what have I done?" I wondered. It was nothing more than a geriatric warehouse.

When we were ushered into a room directly across from the nurses' station, I had another surge of panic. It was ten by ten, the same depressing colour as the hallway. The small window housed an aged, rusty air conditioner and provided a view of a concrete block wall. A bed, a metal table to slide over the bed, a bare bookcase, and the bright overhead light were the only accessories. From the bed Bill would see only the bare, bleak wall and the sad, ugly bookcase. The terrazzo floor was cold and slippery.

"Oh please, God, make our stay here short," I prayed.

As the paramedics moved Bill from the gurney to his new bed I battled the urge to implore them to put him back on and take us home. We shouldn't be here.

The paramedics handed Bill's charts to a nurse and headed down the hallway. The nurse didn't identify herself. Nor did she speak to Bill. Instead she spoke directly to me, as though her new charge was deaf. I was wounded for him, again.

"Mr. MacLeod will be in isolation for a few days, so gowns and gloves will be mandatory. Deposit them in the bin each time you leave the room. Re-gown and glove when you re-enter."

It was a clipped order. Her body language made me think of her as Nurse Sergeant-Major.

"Why?" I asked.

"He is being tested for a contagious bacterial infection, and the results won't be in for a few days."

This was news to me, and both Bill and I were alarmed.

She was referring to MRSA, a hospital-contracted bacteria. I learned later that MRSA stands for Methicillin-resistant Staphylococcus aureus, a pathogen that is resistant to treatment with methicillin, an antibiotic that is effective against most other "staph" infections. It is almost exclusively transmitted by staff. Because of an increase in MRSA worldwide, and in many Canadian health care facilities, testing for this pathogen is recommended, but not always done, in Canadian hospitals.

Bill's first impression of this new place, which I had repeatedly told him would be so great, was of a dull, bleak institution where the only people he would see would be wearing masks and gowns. I felt even greater suspicion about being told I couldn't view the place in advance. Now I realized I should have insisted.

Talking to Bill I tried to reinforce the fact that this was only a stop gap for rehabilitation, but I didn't feel I was giving him much peace of mind.

Late that night, after helping him get settled in, I finally, reluctantly, dragged myself home. The minute I was inside our front door I was hit with a tsunami of anxiety, fear, and sadness. Early that very morning I had been so hopeful, so optimistic, so trusting. Now, guilt stung me like a slap. Had I had let myself be conned?

I paced the floor throughout the long night, obsessing over this new circumstance and feeling betrayed by the system. I hoped Bill was sleeping soundly. The only positive item on my list by five in the morning was that I was a mere five minutes away from him. A small comfort, but it did allow me to be in his room before he woke up.

The first person I met as I stepped out of the dingy elevator in the morning was our family doctor. Dr. Shirriff was a serious man. He looked trim and energetic. At six feet three he could be considered imposing. I guessed him to be in his mid-forties, but his closely cropped fair hair and golf tan gave him a younger appearance. When he smiled he appeared almost light-hearted and casual.

I blurted all the information I thought he needed. "The oncologist came to see us Monday. She sees no need to do chemotherapy at this point. She said there is no evidence in the scans of any malignant disease, so there is nothing to treat. But she was shocked and concerned about Bill's de-conditioned state. We have a lot of rehab work ahead."

Dr. Shirriff looked as though I had just said Bill had enjoyed his trip to Mars. Was that the wife-in-denial look I just saw? He collected the chart from the nurses' station and proceeded into Bill's new accommodations. As he checked Bill over, his first question was, "How did *this* happen?" He was examining the spaces between Bill's thumbs and fingers. The atrophy was disturbing.

"Oh, there's lots of that," I said. "Amazing what two months in bed can do, isn't it?"

My remark was reinforced by what he saw as he continued his examination. Most of Bill's muscles had atrophied. His skin was loose, wasted. Dr. Shirriff talked to Bill, asked him a few questions, and poked and prodded here and there. I was relieved Bill chose to answer him. He didn't always. The doctor said he would be looking into Bill's chart and would see us later.

Fair enough. I was certain once he read the oncology information, we would communicate better.

For the first few days, most of the nurses were friendly and remained patient with my endless questions about the routine and the therapies. There was so much information I needed to share with them so they would understand our goal: to help Bill regain his stamina, energy, and abilities.

"He has progressed a lot already with positive reinforcement, encouragement, and repetitive methods," I told anyone who would listen.

But soon enough, few seemed to really care. They seemed to think I was in denial — or was completely nuts.

9

A FINE MESS

Three days later, the test results were in: no infectious disease. Bill's visitors were grateful they could discard the cumbersome hot gowns and gloves, and Bill seemed relieved to see full faces again.

As days went by, though, I began to realize that our family doctor, this unit, and this hospital had accepted, and expected, a patient they believed was either going to die soon or live out his last days in a nursing home. The notion that he was in their care for rehabilitation was obviously foreign to them.

How could this kind of miscommunication have happened? What had I done? I berated myself constantly but tried not to let my fears show.

Judy came back from Nova Scotia again. I hoped she would at least collect frequent flyer points. She had become my life preserver, encouraging me to carry on as though the staff understood and supported our goals and would get on board soon.

Our first mission, a daunting one, was to improve Bill's room. We tackled the job with gusto. We taped dozens of bright, cheerful cards on the walls, reading each one aloud to Bill. I carted books and plants in from home for the drab bookcase. Once filled with CDs and other personal items, it looked a little less stark. We set up a whiteboard — the same one I had used at KGH — for Bill's schedule, as well as a calendar and a large clock. We placed photos of family and friends and better times directly in his line of sight, with pictures of Jessie Puppy given centre stage.

"This will all be ours again at home soon, Hon," I said. "We just need to stay here long enough to get over this hurdle."

THE PERSON I desperately wanted to meet with, Marg, the physiotherapist, came in on the fourth day. She was the one who would set up the plans for Bill's rehab work. I was already acutely aware it would take incredible work and time to combat Bill's de-conditioned state, so I was anxious for her to get him started on the real road to recovery. We needed her expertise.

She said she needed time to do her own detailed assessment and would meet with me again in a few days.

Judy and I were filled with optimism when we arrived at the lounge a few days later for our follow-up appointment with her — and were totally unprepared for her pronouncement.

She launched into her speech without preamble. "Well, you know, he will never be able to sit up on his own, or stand, and *for sure* he will never walk again, or pee, on his own," she declared.

Pontificated, really. We were stunned. And devastated. I wanted to pummel the woman. "Who the hell is she talking about?" I thought. "She must have skipped Psychology 101, too. What information did she get and from where? Doesn't she realize Bill has had brain surgery and been bedridden for two months?"

I knew anyone taking such a closed, negative position wasn't likely to work for, fight for, or advocate for him. For us.

She explained some simple passive exercises she would set up for him, but her voice indicated it wasn't going to make much difference.

Once she had gathered her papers and left the lounge, I turned to Judy, and said, "*This* is the person who is going to plan his therapy, set the tone, and direct his rehab? God help us."

Thus was laid the foundation for my "screw you" attitude — and my insatiable quest for acquired brain injury education. It was the beginning of my awareness that our health care system had let us down. Badly. My concerns, mistrust, and anxieties continued to grow.

EVERY NEW DAY with Bill was just that, a new day.

Sometimes he was quite alert and talkative, other days somber and sleepy. Sometimes he remembered what this was all about, sometimes not. Sometimes he seemed overwhelmed and unable to process new things. Sometimes he didn't remember staff, other times he did. But he always knew me, his sister, his friends, and his family doctor — although a few times he told me Dr. Mike seemed a little confused!

Some days I noted small physical improvements, other days not. But Bill always remembered our secret message — "I love you." "I love you more." Always whispered.

Welcome to a trip through brain injury.

Most evenings I climbed up onto the bed with him and we pulled the tiny TV over so we could both hear it with the headset. Curled up together we had a refuge from the world, from which we could muse about how awesome it was to just cuddle and be left alone together. Our bear hugs and smooch tests continued, even though there wasn't the same need for the tests. We just really enjoyed them.

Every night I had to force myself to leave the hospital. Whenever I was away from Bill I was lonely, filled with dread, fear, resentment, and frustration. But each morning miraculously brought a renewed drive to make this situation work for him. Every morning we talked about the coming day, and I wrote the information on the whiteboard so he could anticipate what was to come next in his routine.

Meanwhile, I tried to communicate to the staff how important it was to *assist* him, not *do for him*, as much as possible. He still needed coaching for almost everything but was able to do more and more for himself. Repetition of what they called the ADLS (activities of daily living) and his exercises were vital for him to be able to go home. Much of the time I suspected I might as well have been talking to myself.

Several of the nurses did make a big effort to help Bill maximize his abilities and also tried to teach me anything they could. Others learned quickly it was easier to tell me what I wanted to hear. These nurses just carried on with their routines as though they believed he was going to die and I was a little crazy.

I learned very quickly that rehabilitation was not the mandate of this unit, and that the staff were not trained or experienced in brain injury rehab work. Nor did they have neurology experience.

I must have seemed tremendously demanding, arrogant, and suspicious. But then, they didn't know or understand what I had been expecting of them and their unit.

THE PHYSIOTHERAPIST ARRANGED to get a deluxe wheelchair. Finally, Bill would be able to be out of bed. It was shockingly expensive — $5,750 — in large part paid for by the health care system. The good points: Bill could recline in it when he needed a change in position. He could nap in it if he wanted to, and it would enable him to be out of bed much longer, reducing some of the risks I had learned about: of pneumonia, skin breakdown, and other potential setbacks. The bad points: It couldn't be folded and put in the trunk of the car, nor could he propel it by foot. In fact, it did not give him any additional independence, and might even reduce what he already had.

When I raised these questions with Marg I saw that now too familiar wife-in-denial look. Her expression said two things very clearly: Bill and I were never going anywhere in our car, and Bill would never be able to foot-propel it anyway. I resigned myself to knowing at least he could be out of bed and out of his cubicle and get more help exercising.

A day or two later, Judy and I arrived in the morning to discover that Bill's bed was empty. A nurse pointed us to a lounge. We rushed down the hallway, anxious to share this inaugural outing with him. Rounding the corner, we both stopped dead in our tracks.

Bill was slumped in the wheelchair, head hanging down, as if trying to protect himself from the scene before him: Six or seven other inmates were there, as well. Most of them were ancient and in various states of lethargy. The big-screen TV was blaring, and no one else seemed to know it was even turned on. A number of neglected, bedraggled brown plants languished on the windowsills. This was not a lounge. It was reminiscent of a scene from the old Jack Nicholson movie *One Flew Over the Cuckoo's Nest*.

As fast as I could move, I raced my precious husband back to his private room, and then stormed out to speak to the nurse in charge. Through clenched teeth, I said, "Never, never, never is Bill to be taken out of his room again unless someone is going to stay and engage him in something positive."

I knew I was risking further isolation for him, but I also knew in my heart and soul that isolation would be far less damaging to his spirit than those surroundings. He was fifty-six years old, not ninety-six.

OUR FIRST TRIP in his new chair, to the courtyard, was humbling. The designers of this new hospital wing had neglected to include an automatic door, and there was a step right at the doorway. I struggled with the door, the step, and the wheelchair, straining to keep from tipping Bill out of the chair.

I cursed myself. What was I thinking? Maybe it was just too soon to be trying this. Maybe they were right. Maybe, maybe, maybe.

But finally we were out. The patio was quiet and cool, shielded by an umbrella, no one was moaning, and it didn't reek of urine, excrement, and medication. I had brought lunch for us and handed

Bill the sandwich and drink alternately. Meals still took forever, but I could see he was sitting straighter and more balanced. That was very encouraging.

I explained I needed go to the washroom, and raced the fifteen metres across the courtyard. Returning less than three minutes later, I saw Bill hanging over the side of the wheelchair like the straw man in *The Wizard of Oz*. I was horrified. What if I had taken even one more minute? Would he have lost the struggle with gravity?

As I strained to heave him back to an upright position, I heard him say, "Well, this is a fine mess you've gotten us into, Ollie!"

It was an old inside joke of ours. If only I had found it funny. As it was, I berated myself for being incompetent.

Bill loved food and was now eating much better and regaining some weight. He often told me, though, that the food wasn't very good. The master of understatement. As part of my new education I learned an obscure fact: the food budget for long-term care patients is about half the budget for prisoners in our jails.

One day Judy cooked and delivered one of Bill's favourite meals, an authentic salt-fish dinner, While they were both eating, a nurse popped in to investigate the aromas. She was a very big gal, and expressed her personal love for Atlantic cuisine. She lamented not being able to partake. As the hefty backside left the room, Bill looked at us, rolled his eyes, stretched his hands wide, and said, "Oh Good Lord!"

We howled with laughter. Yes, the real Bill was still in there.

Each day we did at least two exercise sessions, sometimes three. Doing leg lifts, knee bends, and arm stretches, using hand weights, and rolling side to side — all this was increasing his muscle strength and flexibility. It was encouraging and provided purpose to the days, and I regretted not starting these activities and passive exercises from day one in the regional hospital. Maybe that would have staved off at least some of the muscle atrophy and balance problems.

PART TWO

*FROM FEAR
TO ANGER*

10

SEEKING BALANCE

THE PHYSIOTHERAPIST OR ONE of her assistants worked with Bill as often as possible, but it was only a couple of times a week. One of the assistants took a special interest in him. Tracey was a godsend. While she worked with him at sitting on the bedside to improve his balance, she also got creative. She asked Bill to look up at the ceiling and point out articles such as the curtain rod, the light fixture, or the doorframe. This required him to lean forward and backward, and turn to one side or the other.

I stuck coloured letters and numbers all over his room, even on the ceiling, and Tracey asked him to read out certain ones or pick out a particular picture. Bill talked to her more than anyone else on staff. On the days I was away at work she left messages on the board for us about Bill's accomplishments.

Tracey seemed to be the only one who believed he had real potential. After only a few weeks, though, despite Bill's evident improvements, she was told to limit her time with us. The priority of the physiotherapy staff was acute care patients.

I was outraged, and asked myself why they wouldn't want Bill out as fast as possible, too; why he should be less of a priority.

As days turned into weeks, Bill made great strides in balance and posture. He was eating, shaving, brushing his teeth, brushing his hair, and much more. He was interacting with many of the staff, especially those who showed genuine interest in him.

I pleaded with the nurses to help him get dressed in real clothes when I was at work.

"He's a military man who is proud of being impeccably groomed and dressed," I said. "This is part of his spirit. This is important."

Some of the staff did try their best, but evidently others didn't see the point.

Small battles erupted every time I arrived and found Bill wearing a diaper. Yes, it was time consuming to help a patient dress in regular clothes as opposed to a diaper and hospital gown, but I believed the whole person is important. Skin breakdown and infections are by-products of these labour-saving diapers, but worse, they make patients feel debilitated and hopeless. Weren't nurses supposed to do everything possible to prevent new problems? Wasn't part of their job to keep their patients' confidence and hope alive? Wasn't it obvious to them that a sad mind and spirit would impede progress?

Dr. Shirriff agreed I could take our puppy Jessie to visit whenever I wanted. She made Bill laugh when she leaped all over him on the bed and licked his face. He threw toys onto the floor for her to retrieve. It was always a joyful reunion.

My sister Brenda and some close friends tried to visit Bill on Thursdays and Fridays when I couldn't be there. They often arrived bearing goodies. This alleviated a huge concern for me about going to work and having to leave him for long periods of time, uncertain how his day would be spent. On some level I was always worried he would be neglected.

11

"THE RIGHT THING"

That month I started a journal so we could keep track of Bill's activities, improvements, and gaps. Keeping this journal soon became my main source of encouragement, and I shared information from it with anyone on staff who would listen. Bill was still a whole person: a kind, thoughtful, decent man, full of determination. I continued to believe and remind him daily we would have our life (albeit a different life) back soon.

That spring I learned of an Acquired Brain Injury conference in Peterborough, Ontario, focusing on rehabilitation. I attended, soaking up the information and ideas. I learned about the benefits of taking photos to remind Bill who the staff members were, to help him keep track of the endless rotation of faces. The importance of continuity, consistency, and repetition were all emphasized. I learned about identity mapping: Helping Bill relearn his self-image would require a biography and pictures of his life for the people who would be working with him. I also learned it often took a minimum of seeing or repeating something four times for it to "click." I felt encouraged that we were working in the right direction.

But I was also even more convinced my husband was in a very unsuitable place.

In the evenings we still curled up together on his bed and read the papers or just talked. This physical contact was the best part of my day. Feeling those strong hands holding me, stroking my head and rubbing my back reinforced my confidence in our unique relationship. We shared so much love for and trust in each other. We couldn't leave it to others to decide our future.

One afternoon in the middle of May, while I attended to "other life" stuff, Brenda went to spend time with Bill. She took fresh strawberry tarts, strawberries being one of the very few fruits Bill wasn't allergic to.

"Should we eat these right away, Bill?" she asked.

"Well, they won't be much good in January," he replied.

She was still laughing, hours later, describing his impish grin.

Realizing I couldn't do everything myself and the staff truly didn't have the time Bill's rehabilitation required, I started a search for volunteers who would be willing to come into the hospital. I wrote letters to every service club and church group in our region. Nothing. I called all the agencies I thought connected volunteers with people needing their services. Nothing.

Finally one call led to a contact at the Regional Community Brain Injury Services office in Belleville. RCBIS provides services to people with brain injuries and related issues in the community where they live. Wendy Haddrall, the woman I spoke to, sounded very concerned by our story and made an appointment to come to see us. I felt I had finally found someone who would help me to help and advocate for Bill.

"Thank you, God," I prayed.

Wendy, a counsellor, explained that her organization's purpose was to support people with brain injuries, mainly those at home or in group homes. The office she worked at in Belleville was a satellite of the main office in Kingston. Wendy's background in Behavioural Sciences and her understanding of the practical problems faced by people with brain injuries was apparent. She had a wealth of knowledge about issues like Bill's and a multitude of practical suggestions and information.

Over the following few weeks, she helped me stay on track and took the time to get to know Bill as well as his case. Who he had been before all this change was very important to her, and she taught me how to use that information to help him.

I sent letters to our political representatives at all levels, questioning the lack of facilities for a complicated patient like Bill, with or without acquired brain injury, and asking for their help. I explained how desperate we were. Of the three people I wrote to, one didn't even respond, one said, "Health care isn't a federal issue," and the other said, "Yes, we are aware that there are glitches in the system, and I am sorry. But I do wish you good luck."

My fears were growing, but now my anger outranked them. How dare that provincial official call my husband's circumstance, or the problems of anyone else's loved one, a *glitch*. I vowed I would never vote for any of these people again.

THE MONTHS IN Complex Continuing Care were fraught with many ups and downs. Bill made progress, and then slid back a little, made more progress, and slid a little. This was due partly to brain injury and partly to medical mistakes: oversights, medications given incorrectly or at the wrong times, incorrect information. These things kept me on edge. I never knew whether to chalk them up to lack of staff or knowledge. Or both.

Bill developed several urinary tract infections while we there, which usually triggered short bouts of seizures. I still didn't understand why he had been on a catheter all this time. Catheters make things convenient for the nurses but frequently cause other problems. In Bill's case, they caused infections, and infections very often triggered seizures.

Slowly, his muscles were getting stronger and his flexibility and balance were improving. His voice was stronger and the swallowing issues had disappeared. But significant fatigue and "moon face," two of the known side effects of taking Decadron, still plagued him. I continued to badger the staff for this drug to be reassessed, even presenting them with a page of facts about its side effects.

Finally, one day near the end of May, I got into a heated discussion with Dr. Shirriff. After raising the question of this drug and its side effects with him again, he said, "I wouldn't be comfortable changing this medication without input from Dr. Ellis."

"Well, go use the goddamn phone," was my not very gracious answer.

He did, and the very next day, voilà, the slow weaning process began. Within a few days, Bill was more energetic, more engaged, and dozing far less. His response confirmed my suspicion that this drug was at the root of many of his problems.

I recalled my many conversations with staff at Kingston General about this drug, when I was first aware that it could be problematic, causing muscle weakness, confusion, lethargy, inability to stay with a thought process, short-term memory loss, and a host of other side effects. It seemed I had been the only one to make the connection. I began to question myself for not taking this up directly a second time with Dr. Ellis back then.

Miscommunication was still one of our greatest adversaries.

It also appeared to me that no one was actually reading Bill's chart, except perhaps its first page. While at work every Thursday and Friday, I was consumed with worry. Would the staff recognize the signs of a problem? Would the nurses help him or just do everything for him to save time? Would they remind him I was at work, to ease his mind? Would they engage him in conversation and treat him as a person? What new issues would crop up while I was gone?

One day a potential miracle came our way. Terri Cjaika, woman from the Chedoke Rehabilitation Centre in Hamilton, about two and a half hours west of Trenton, was coming to assess another patient, and the charge nurse had asked if she could see Bill as well. I was grateful to this nurse manager, particularly as we didn't have a good rapport. Chedoke was the very place Walter Gretzky had been for rehabilitation. I was filled with hope. Surely this person would recognize Bill's potential, understand his progress, and not be discouraged by his ups and downs. I prayed for the help he needed and deserved.

When Terri came to meet Bill she asked him a few questions, most of which he ignored. He rarely interacted well with people he didn't know. I guessed that, rather than appear odd, he just refrained from responding. It was very rare that he didn't talk to me, and others he knew, but strangers? Often he simply avoided them in his own way.

In the end, the answer was, "No, he isn't suitable for the program."

I was devastated to find out that the patient she was originally there to see, who was dramatically less functional than Bill, *was* accepted. Then I felt horribly guilty for resenting him.

No one had told me their criteria required a patient to be medically stable for three months before being considered. The question loomed in my mind: How would Bill ever get medically stable here, with so little suitable help and so many issues popping up all the time? Here where his spirit was slowly being crushed like rocks into powder? God help us.

ONE FRIDAY NIGHT in mid-July, during the one-hundred-and-fifty-kilometre trek home from Toronto, I was overcome with a feeling of fear and dread. Something was very wrong. I drove directly to the hospital. In his room, I discovered Bill absolutely vibrating in the bed, and in a high fever. I asked the nurse what time she had given him the injection. He had been in this state for several hours according to her verbal report, but she hadn't administered the drug for seizures.

"These aren't seizures; they are tremors," she said defensively.

I gave her a very rude, very short course on how to distinguish seizures from tremors and insisted she get a real doctor, and quickly. I asked for mountains of ice, a fan, and lots of towels. The air conditioner was barely cooling the room, and Bill needed his body temperature brought down quickly. How odd it was that I was the one directing this treatment.

When a doctor finally appeared, one of his first questions was, "Why is he here instead of in Acute Care?"

The same question had crossed my mind. After checking Bill, and determining the steps to proceed, he asked me to step outside the room with him.

"Mrs. MacLeod, do you have a DNR order for your husband?"

"What's that?"

"Do Not Resuscitate. I don't think your husband has more than a couple of weeks left. You need to do the right thing for him."

My heart pounded in my ears. I thought I might vomit. I used all my energy to keep from slapping him. He had come to this prognosis after spending fewer than eight minutes in the room with Bill? I wondered if he had even read any part of Bill's chart.

I explained we'd been through these setbacks before, usually stemming from an infection not yet found, and how this often led to seizures. I asked him to come back to see Bill in a few days when the patient had rebounded again. He agreed to do that but in exchange asked me to think seriously about his advice. I agreed. Neither of us followed through.

OUR ONLY REAL HOPE

A™ THAT PRECISE MOMENT, I realized Bill would be safer at home with me than in Complex Continuing Care. We were in the wrong place.

Within a few days, with the infection found and treated, Bill was back to his new normal. I'd had plenty of time to think about our experience in this institution. Enough was enough. I discussed my thoughts with him.

"Want to go home?" I asked.

"Of course!"

"Do you believe we can we do this together?"

"Of course!"

"Would you like to pick a date?"

"Tomorrow?"

"That might be a little too soon, Hon. There are some things I need to set up first. How about in two weeks?"

"Done."

I wrote "Going home July 26/2003" on the whiteboard and circled the date on the calendar. I knew now this was our only hope, but, still, my anxiety and fears kicked up another notch.

The decision to go home was so right, but it was also terrifying. I had learned a lot, but I also knew how much I didn't know. I hadn't resolved the details about how I would manage, about who would stay with him when I went to work. The social workers in both hospitals said Bill could get only two hours a day of home care. Sixty hours a month was the mandate then of the province's Community Care Access Centres system. I would have to figure something out.

But first things first.

Judy and her husband, Andy, flew in from Nova Scotia to help me prepare our home for this new phase. A contractor removed two walls and a bathtub, converting what had been a guest room and bathroom into one large multipurpose room. It was adjacent to our family room. Fortunately, our home had a main floor entry, and lots of space on the first level, plus patio doors to the yard. Now Bill's view would be of our home, our garden, and our puppy playing. A definite step in the right direction if quality of life is the priority.

The carpeting was too thick to be safe, so it had to go. We replaced it with commercial grade. It was ugly but would be safer for using the mechanical lift and would allow Bill to move his wheelchair around by himself. I hoped the day would come when everything could be turned back into normal rooms, but for now safer was better.

Next came the equipment question. Home care services would provide a bed and table and a couple of smaller items for one month only. Bill's recovery was clearly going to take a lot longer than one month, so, with Judy's help, I ordered an electric bed, which Bill would be able to adjust himself whenever he wanted; a mechanical lift; a shower chair; and a few other essentials.

When I sat down and looked at the amount of money I had just spent, I was horrified. Cost of equipment: $9,600. The contractor's bill: $4,500. Carpeting: $2,000.

But our new setup was perfect. Putting the hospital bed and a single bed side by side in our former family room created a king-sized bed. Our new bedroom had a stereo, a TV, a gas fireplace, a lovely view, and even the usual place for the Christmas tree later. Friends built a low ramp for the front entry so the few inches of rise would be easier for me to maneuver. I reflected again and again on how fortunate we were to have a home that was so easily converted.

The family room opened onto a screened porch Bill had built for me years before. The porch had two doors leading to decks on each side, one in a private, peaceful shade garden, the other in a bright, sunny area with beds of colourful plants and flowering shrubs. Our lawn and gardens were quite beautiful, the result of many seasons of shared work and pleasure. We would be able to spend many, many peaceful hours there, throwing toys for Jessie and soaking in the sense of home.

A shower base replaced the bathtub. Our neighbour Al constructed two low ramps, one for inside and one for outside the shower. The trip into the shower would be a relatively smooth up and over. The first few times it was anything but simple, but eventually we mastered it.

All these changes evoked a multitude of emotions in me. I was sad to see our lovely home, and the essence of our life together, so changed. But I was elated that we would finally be together all the time in our own comfortable fortress. Here we could continue our life and protect each other from the never-ending negative attitudes. Those had already done enough damage.

My unspoken questions still loomed like monsters, though. "What if the professionals are right and we can't do it? But unless we try, how will we ever know?"

I acknowledged to myself, but no one else, "The nursing homes are not likely to disappear if I am wrong."

The hospital administration, our family doctor, and some staff were concerned about and even angry at my decision to take Bill home. Nearly every conversation about our decision was laced with negative opinions.

The Community Care Access Centre liaison manager said, "Catherine, do you not understand your husband has brain cancer?"

"Actually, right now he does not. According to the most recent CT scan and his oncologist, and I am quoting, 'There is no residual disease.' So, unless and until that changes, you need to stop treating him as if he does. And if that changes, chemo is still an option."

Dr. Shirriff said, "Catherine, you are making a huge mistake. You can't possibly manage Bill at home on your own. If you take him out of here, you can't reasonably expect much help later."

I retaliated with a question: "What part of 'for better and for worse' did you and your wife not sign on for?"

I did not want to argue with or alienate him, sensing he could be a formidable adversary. I knew he was truly concerned about Bill, but I realized he simply could not see any other options for us. That he didn't understand us, our commitment, or our desperation.

Some of the staff did offer tremendous encouragement, saying, "Get him out of here as fast as you can." Those who supported our decision also took the time to give us as much instruction as possible.

I soon developed a pat answer for those who didn't: "If you won't help us do this, will you at least get the hell out of our way?"

Bill was delighted and excited about getting home, and I was very, very grateful. And very, very scared. In fact I was petrified. My questions and concerns mushroomed. I knew I couldn't leave him alone while I went to work, and that two hours a day of home care wouldn't suffice. But I was more afraid of leaving him in this warehouse.

Several days before Bill was to leave the hospital, I met with Dr. Shirriff in his office, armed with questions about what to do at home. As I proceeded through the nuts and bolts of my concerns, I sensed he was edgy, or angry, or both. Suddenly I felt very intimidated. Having already overrun my appointment time, I didn't ask the last, most important question on my list: "What do I do in a crisis?"

WE WERE EXCITED about getting home and looking forward to so many things, including throwing toys for Jessie again. She would be a great diversion for Bill and would also benefit from the attention. She had missed Bill so much, and looked so pathetic each time I left to go to the hospital without her. I could see she was suffering right along with me. My grief about losing the life we had been blessed with was undeniable. That I couldn't share this with the only person on earth who would truly understand was unbearable. But I needed to stay focused on our immediate concerns.

Truly at the eleventh hour, a day before we were to head for home, I learned Bill could, in fact, get extra home care. Personal support workers (PSWs) and nurses could be there the two days each week that I was at work. With the costs mounting, and beginning to matter, I was relieved that I could continue my work. It occurred to me it would be selfish and callous to hope for enough help to return to work full-time. I understood the system couldn't provide everything.

One step at a time, though. We'd be sleeping together in our own bed, in our own home, with Jessie. Living our life together. Bill and I were frantic with excitement, like little kids on Christmas Eve. Could there be a better therapy on earth?

Finally, the homecoming I'd promised. Saying goodbye to the Complex Continuing Care unit on that morning of July 26 was easy. The card I left at the desk read:

> *To those of you who encouraged me that I am doing the right thing, I am very grateful. To those who came to understand that I was simply advocating for a better quality of life for my partner, thank you. To those of you who were able to see Bill as a whole person with real potential and deserving of a real chance, thank you.*

I shed no tears leaving the warehouse.

13

HOME AGAIN

On july 26, 2003, five months and ten days since Bill's second post-surgery return to hospital, we were finally home together. As the driver brought Bill out of the wheelchair transport van in our driveway, joy, gratitude, love, and trepidation bubbled up inside me.

Judy and Andy were at the door to welcome Bill home, but as soon as Jessie spotted him she darted past them and launched herself onto his lap, licking and kissing him and burrowing into his body. Bill gave out a hearty laugh, rubbing her fur with glee.

Up the low ramp, through the doorway, and right into our new living area we rolled. Bill looked bemused. Taking in the changes in our décor, he remarked, "This is different. Hmmm."

I rolled his wheelchair across the room to the sliding door so he could see the backyard.

"Wow! Everything is so alive! Look at our lilies!" he said.

Our gardens were stunning that July, full and lush, with a kaleidoscope of colour, as if the plants too had made extra effort to welcome Bill home.

Throughout the day I could see he still didn't fully understand or remember his new limitations. Fortunately the wheelchair belt prevented him from trying to stand up when he wanted to take a walk outside.

"Hon, right now your legs are just not strong enough for you to walk, but that will come. You are going to have to do a lot of exercises to build your muscles back up. We'll work on them together. Okay?"

"Okey dokey," he said. Always obliging.

Not recognizing your own deficiencies is *not* a good thing in a neurology or rehab assessment, but for us, especially now that we were home, Bill's lack of awareness of the changes in himself kept him from becoming frustrated, angry, or discouraged. He lived almost exclusively in the present. I tried to do so, too; the present was all we had. This would be the start of the (albeit amateur) rehabilitation he had been denied. Until now. I blessed those patient care assistants at the Kingston General for all they had taught me.

Judy cooked Bill's favourite maritime dinner, salt beef and cabbage, to celebrate this miraculous homecoming — the homecoming that supposedly was impossible.

Sleeping together in our own bed, in our own home, after nearly six months, was glorious. As we stretched out, Jessie claimed her usual place right between us. I closed my eyes, committing this experience to memory: The luxury of our skin touching; the familiar, subtle smell of Bill's aftershave; the whisper of his gentle breathing; the protection of his arms wrapping me into him. Sleeping together like two old spoons was a gift. This was why I had fought so hard. This was *our life*.

THE VERY NEXT day a Home Care case manager from the Community Care Access Centre for our area called and asked if she could meet us both that afternoon to assess Bill and his needs. CCACs, part of Ontario's Ministry of Health, hire the services of nurses, personal support workers, therapists, and social workers from service agencies like Red Cross, Paramed, and the Victoria Order of Nurses to care for people in their community.

I sensed immediately that Linda, a former nurse, was compassionate and caring.

She explained the details about home care services as they pertained to Bill.

"Home Care can provide a registered practical nurse for eight-hour shifts on Thursdays and Fridays. The nursing hours come from a different program. They're separate from the sixty hours of personal support care in the regular program, and some of those PSW hours can be used to cover the remaining hours when you'll be at work."

As Linda talked, the little devil on my shoulder whispered, "If you had known this extra help was possible, Cath, would you ever have left him in that warehouse for all those months?" I shushed it.

Bill slept peacefully through most of the conversation. I didn't ask any questions about the separate program the nurses would come from. It was a miracle that my biggest concern about going to work had been answered. I thought that was all I needed to know.

Linda and I worked out a schedule for the first month. A personal support worker would come for an hour in the morning and an hour in the evening, Saturday to Wednesday, to help Bill with hygiene, dressing, and undressing, and a PSW would replace the nurse and stay until I got home from work the other two nights. The case manager also arranged for a registered nurse to come to assess Bill's medical needs. A physiotherapist, an occupational therapist, and a speech therapist were scheduled to do their own assessments within two weeks.

We talked about specific needs. Bill had come home with an indwelling catheter to void urine. Emptying it and recording the output was so simple, anyone could do it. I had, many times.

Drawing blood from the "pick" line (a tube installed directly into a vein for long-term use) would require a short nursing visit every other day initially. I hoped it would be removed soon.

I was very comfortable being direct with Linda. I shared my frustration about the lack of rehabilitation available to Bill.

"My main objective," I told her, "is to do whatever we can to help him move forward by keeping him engaged, following the exercise plan, and making sure he gets the necessary food, drink, and rest. He's doing very well on his own schedule. It will be so much better here."

The schedule was prominently displayed on one wall for Bill's benefit, and I had already drafted a small book of details the home care staff would need to know concerning his routine and activities from first thing in the morning to the evening.

"Linda, the most important thing is Bill doing rehabilitation, finally. Thank you."

Theresa, the nurse who would do ongoing assessments of his medical status, quickly established an excellent rapport with both of us. She was knowledgeable, helpful, and capable, and I trusted her opinions almost immediately. Bill liked her, and she was genuinely interested in him.

Adjusting to strangers coming in and out of our home, though, was more nerve-wracking than I had anticipated. I was forever saying, "Please go slower, please be gentle, please let Bill do that for himself, be patient, please don't answer the question for him," and more. Our months of establishing a repetitive way of doing things had worked so well for him. Each new person had to learn the way he already did things.

My first experience with shift nursing was unnerving. Naturally I was anxious and afraid of leaving Bill in the care of a complete stranger, whose skills, ideas, and attitudes were as yet unknown to me. Jennifer, the young registered practical nurse who arrived to cover my first day back to work, appeared to listen only half-heartedly. My commentary on Bill's care, his schedule, and how to enable him seemed to be of little interest to her. I explained our rehab plan and our goals, trying to be clear and concise. I left the book I had created, now called *Bill's Home Care Book*, for her to read during her eight-hour shifts.

I wrestled with my feeling of unease, telling myself, as I drove to Toronto. "For God's sake, Cath, she's an RPN. She'll know how to help him. She will keep him safe. Nancy, the PSW, takes over at three-thirty. They'll each do the head-to-toe bathing and help him with meals and exercises. If they see anything odd, they'll tell you. Be grateful. Have a little faith."

Two weeks later, though, I started to notice that Bill seemed to regress during the days I was at work. I had tried to ignore the little voice in my head. It had started out subtle as a soft summer breeze, just a little whisper. But it had grown into a howling wind.

There was something I just couldn't quite put my finger on. During week three I set up a test. I drew a large red X on the top of Bill's right foot before putting his socks on him in the morning. Returning from work fifteen hours later, I removed the sock.

"Surprise!" I muttered. The X was still there. I brooded about it, but left the scarlet letter there. When I arrived home the next night, there was a different issue to digest.

"I got here a little early and Bill was tied in his chair with a bedsheet," Nancy said. "Jennifer said she was worried that he would try to get out of the chair."

The irony of Jennifer's concern was that Bill couldn't have gotten out of the chair if his life had depended on it. I had spent much of my time encouraging him to keep working on that, knowing it helped strengthen his muscles. I wondered, if the nurse's concern was in fact genuine, why she hadn't just tilted the chair back or put the tray on it in front of him. My main concern, though, was the psychological damage of being tied into a chair.

As soon we were alone I whipped off Bill's right sock. Yep, the big red X was still there. I struggled with my question: How could two people, each working a shift each day over two days, both give

Bill a head-to-toe bed bath, a thorough skin check, and an application of foot cream and not remove the big red X? Neither of them had asked me why it was there. I could only assume they had not seen it.

The next Thursday (I now loathed Thursdays) when the nurse arrived, I broached my concerns. First, I explained to Jennifer about the big red X that had still been there at bedtime the previous Friday night.

Before she could answer, I said, "My other concern is more serious. Did you tie Bill in his chair with a bedsheet? And if you did, I need to understand why."

In just moments her pretty features went from soft white to stormy black. Her eyes were wide and glaring.

"You were trying to trap me, weren't you?" she yelled. "You're trying to make trouble for me. The PSW should have done his feet! He was trying all day to get out of the chair. He said he could get up. He should be in a bed, not in a chair."

I tried a different tack. I asked her to sit in the wheelchair. I tilted it to Bill's normal position.

"See if you can get out of the chair, Jennifer, and really focus on the coordination and strength it takes."

She couldn't get out.

"I was not trying to trap you, Jennifer. Nor the PSW. It is my responsibility to look out for Bill, both his physical and his mental well-being. It is my job to protect him. That is all I was trying to do by asking you directly."

I couldn't get Jennifer's wild eyes out of my mind, and during my subsequent call to the case manager I insisted that the agency never send her to our home again.

"Bill needs people who won't get frustrated with him and will be of a mindset to really work with us," I said. "This isn't a reading lounge. It's not babysitting. He needs to work toward improvement. He can't be tied in a chair. That's inappropriate, cruel, and, in case this nurse doesn't know, also against the law!"

Weeks later I learned that Jennifer had subsequently been placed with an elderly Alzheimer's patient, alone in the patient's home.

In the first few weeks, always racing to be ready for someone, I found it more stressful having help for two one-hour periods a day than having none. I cancelled the Saturday to Wednesday support. This made it easier for Bill and me to improve our routines, have more privacy, and share tasks.

AS BILL'S STAMINA improved, his regimen changed. He was now actively participating in washing, brushing his teeth, shaving, and getting dressed. Though he still needed constant reminders about what should come next, he was making measurable and notable progress. Morning, noon, and night we shared our "I love yous" and our smooch test. That made everything worthwhile.

Gradually we modified the schedule as we encountered successes and setbacks. I was delighted to have time, after the day's routine, to sit on the deck, listen to music, and watch man and dog. Bill's fine-motor skills were improving dramatically as he repeated the exercise of sneaking Jessie tiny treats. He tried to hide this from me, clearly remembering I didn't think she should be hand fed. That was real cognitive progress! Painstakingly breaking up a small piece of meat, or a cracker, or a piece of cheese into smaller segments, he'd reach down with the goodies. If he forgot to open his fingers for her to take the treat, she'd whine to get his attention.

Bill in turn would admonish her, saying, "Shhhhh, your mom won't be happy."

14

THE NEW BILL

OUR NEED FOR CONTACT and involvement with family and friends won out over my anguish about exposing the *new* Bill to others. Controlled visiting was imperative, because someone might inadvertently bring along a bug or virus; nothing could be done on a drop-in basis any more. Planning and adjusting to accommodate social visits was well worth the effort, though, and I knew it would get easier as Bill's progress brought him back closer to his old self.

During those first weeks we had some great company. Earl and Joyce would come by for coffee and bring maple donuts. My Aunt Lorraine and my cousin Susan drove from Toronto, and catered a delightful lunch to boot. Al and Brenda drove the one hundred and twenty-five kilometres from their home in Ajax to help make this monumental change feel at least a little bit normal.

When my sister Brenda was faced with an unexpected move, we talked it over and she (and her cat) came to stay with us for a few months until she could find a new home. It would help her and would certainly be a great benefit to me, since she was quite comfortable spending time with Bill.

As Bill talked more and became more engaged in our life again, his fatigue was lessening. As weeks passed, the steroid slowly left his system, taking the "moon face" with it. He was beginning to feel and look more like his handsome old self. And we were making progress together. At home.

Sadly, the physiotherapist from the Community Care Access Centre was a tremendous disappointment. After doing her assessment, she merely copied the exercise plan from the physiotherapist at Trenton Hospital. No changes.

I thought, "This person is going to train the home care staff to do physiotherapy work with Bill? Oh shit."

The occupational and speech therapists, conversely, were knowledgeable and encouraging, providing positive information and helpful ideas. They interacted with Bill enthusiastically and were most willing to share information and make recommendations for us to work on.

There were daily changes. Most good. Some not. And another problem had evolved. Nearly every week brought different nurses and different support workers. I should have asked Linda more questions at the beginning, but scheduling to get the same people consistently seemed impossible, and it was a daunting task to get each new person oriented and up to speed about Bill in the fifteen or twenty minutes before I left for work. Some clearly didn't see why these details mattered and seemed confused by my expectations. I was stunned and alarmed when staff who couldn't use the mechanical lift were sent to work eight-hour shifts with Bill. There was no other way to get Bill into his chair.

We seemed to have so many needs that couldn't be filled by agency staff, and I wondered why the agencies scheduled so many people who couldn't meet Bill's needs. Didn't they match staff skills to patient needs? Eventually I realized that staff often either weren't allowed to do certain things due to liability concerns or simply weren't capable.

BILL'S HOME CARE BOOK continued to evolve. It was a real "getting to know Bill inside-out" book, containing his daily schedule, a journal sheet for Bill to check off as he did things, and instructions such as don't tuck the sheets in, his skin gets raw; don't put more than one pillow under his head, he's getting round-shouldered; and don't give him any food other than what I have prepared because of allergies. I added new information as needed, but also sensed that many of the details seemed ridiculous to many of the people providing care. I could only hope and trust they were, in fact, being diligent.

I always had great peace of mind when Theresa, the nurse, was with Bill, however. And fortunately one of the PSWs, Laurie, also stood out from the rest. She was competent, willing to learn Bill's ways, and she brought some laughter to his evenings. I was effusive in telling the case manager what a help these two women were for both of us.

Several times each day, five days a week, Bill and I worked on an exercise in which he just sat on the edge of the bed unsupported. Initially he could manage only ten seconds, but daily his endurance improved: thirty seconds, then forty, then fifty. Finally, he could sit unsupported for sixty seconds. Within two weeks he was sitting for ten minutes without support.

Every day we did exercises with different-sized balls, passing them back and forth, pushing them up and down, and rolling them on the bed. He graduated to leg lifts and leaning forward and backward. Reaching up a few inches higher every day was progress. Every one of these activities contributed to his ability to shave himself, brush his own hair, and live his life better and better. More independence. More encouragement.

Not every day was splendid, though. Some were very disappointing. On those days we tried to forge ahead and do whatever we could anyway, believing tomorrow would be better. Up, down, up, down was the seesaw of home rehabilitation. But each time we got past a rough spot, I was elated. Bill was making progress, and we had our life.

15

THE NEWEST ASSAULT

ON THE THURSDAY BEFORE Labour Day 2003, a new crisis struck.

Waking up, I felt something akin to earthquake aftershocks. Bill's whole body was vibrating. I was pretty sure he was having a low-grade seizure, but I had no idea what to do. I berated myself for not asking Dr. Shirriff, way back in July, before we left the hospital, what I should do in the case of seizures.

Knowing Dr. Shirriff did his rounds early in the morning I called the hospital and begged the charge nurse to get a message to him.

"Just tell him Bill is in trouble," I said.

The doctor returned my call within minutes.

I described what I was seeing, answering his questions as calmly and concisely as I could.

"I am pretty sure these are seizures," I said. "Do you think the home care nurse could give him the Valium injection when she arrives?"

The doctor, trying to make an over-the-phone diagnosis and recommendation, said, "Those can be very tricky, and I am not sure she would be experienced at this."

"Could I give him an extra Dilantin pill to see if that will stop the seizure?"

"Okay, that is worth trying. Keep me posted, please."

When Theresa arrived I gave Bill the crushed pills, plus the extra dose, in yogurt. I prayed this would quiet the seizures.

My business was suffering these days, and I was always torn between it and Bill. Go? Stay? Being self-employed was a serious drawback in our current circumstances. As I left for work that day, I hoped and prayed everything would be fine.

Ninety minutes later, my cell phone rang. It was Theresa, who said, "I thought Bill was choking on the pill mixture. I've spoken to Dr. Shirriff and I've called an ambulance."

I trusted her but prayed she had made the right call.

I took one minute to explain to colleagues that I couldn't stay at work and headed for the Trenton hospital, driving as if I was in the Grand Prix. For the first time in my life I *wanted* to get caught speeding; I was certain it would gain me a police escort the rest of the way.

My entry to the ER cubicle housing Bill is engraved in my memory forever. It was a large room, yet it was crowded. Big, bright overhead lights like an operating room. Monitors beeping and buzzing. Carts full of equipment. Several doctors, several nurses. Bill, on a stretcher, with a breathing apparatus. Wires and tubes everywhere. It was worse than I had expected. Someone tried to get me out of the room but I couldn't be budged. A doctor told me that inserting the tube to help Bill breathe hadn't gone well, and that other concerns were surfacing.

Suddenly, Dr. Shirriff bounded into the already crowded space. His arrival alarmed me more. He should have been in his office tending to patients. He conferred with the group crowded around the stretcher, then came over to me.

"Catherine, Bill needs to go to Kingston General by ambulance," he said. "A nurse will go with him."

Minutes later I realized he was riding with Bill, too. Now I truly understood the gravity of the situation.

At Kingston General, the paramedics raced Bill inside, and Dr. Shirriff and the nurse followed the gurney to the intensive care unit. I paced outside the solid ICU doors praying and begging God and the universe to save my husband again.

After a very long time, Dr. Shirriff reappeared. He looked much less intense now; the furrows on his forehead had receded. He told me he was confident Bill was going to be okay.

"The seizures are abating. Looks like another urinary tract infection. The doctor in the intensive care unit will get him started on an antibiotic. That should do the trick. They're going to keep him for a bit, but he *is* safe."

I wished I could ask him to stay because I didn't want to be here alone if anything *else* went wrong, but I couldn't ask for more than he had already done.

In the intensive care unit I again felt I was in a vacuum. All the monitors and equipment still unnerved me. The indwelling catheter and IV lines were essential, but daunting. I was filled with worry and angst and feelings of uselessness. Again I talked to an unconscious Bill.

"This is only a precaution, and it's my fault, and I'm so, so sorry, and I love you so much."

When the doctor came out he said, "Mrs. MacLeod, there is a possibility that your husband has meningitis. I need to do a spinal tap to confirm or rule it out. I will need your permission."

I recalled we had been through this before. For whatever reason, something about Bill's neck and throat had previously raised this concern. I went back and forth between instinct and logic, thinking, "No, don't do it. He doesn't have that. But what if? What do you know? If he has it and you don't let them find it, something that could have been easily treated could just as easily be fatal."

Finally I gave consent, hoping it was the right decision.

The first concern was the blood thinner Bill was taking. They needed to stop giving him the drug and give him frozen plasma before they could do the test. It actually took two days to get this all done. An eternity to me. "What if he does have meningitis? Is this time loss a serious concern?" There I was, again, with my endless badgering and questions and fear.

The test result was negative, and Bill was moved to recover in a regular room. Thank you, God, again. This time he was given a private room at the end of the hall, farther from the nursing station, but it was peaceful. I was surprised and grateful to learn that Dr. Ellis would be overseeing Bill this time.

On day three, Tuesday, September 2, the neurosurgeon visited and, as usual, spoke directly to Bill, which I always appreciated.

"Well, Bill, you don't have anything you shouldn't have as far as we can tell, but there's a very slight chance you might have another blood clot. We need to get an ultrasound done, just in case. I just want to be absolutely sure you don't have one before we let you go."

Bill agreed it was a wise choice, and the test was done.

Later Dr. Ellis came in himself to say, "Yep, there is a clot, Bill. In fact, there are three, and they're quite large. It's time to drag out the big guns, the clot buster drugs."

It was scary information, but it sounded better coming from him — calm, clear, and direct as usual.

The important thing was to get him on the "wonder drug" and get the clots dissolving. We waited.

When Dr. Ellis surfaced the next morning, it was to recount a strange event.

"Through the night Bill's hemoglobin count suddenly dropped to a critical level. I ordered a CT scan fully expecting to find a major bleed either in the abdomen or into it. It wasn't there. I'm not sure what to make of it, so I have asked for a hematology consult."

Oddly, I appreciated his saying he didn't know something. I was confident he would do his best to find out. A brain surgeon who didn't think he was God!

He came back to see us later with the findings. I was thankful that he always kept us up to date.

"Well, it seems Bill is one of maybe a half million people who have a bizarre reaction to this drug. Effectively, it makes the blood cells disintegrate, which is why they can't be found. The good news is that there is another drug we can use."

He sounded fascinated by this new piece of knowledge. I was just grateful.

"Good. How soon can we go home?" I asked.

"Be patient. This is going to take some time," the doctor admonished, but gently.

Hours turned into days, days into weeks.

This newest assault brought more issues for his body and brain. Daily, Bill seemed to be regressing, some days staying awake for only a few hours. Many days he was too tired and too weak to participate even in the simplest of things. This time, though, I knew enough to keep up the passive exercising of his muscles, and to keep up the mental activity. He was losing ground, though, and I was feeling disheartened.

Dr. Ellis decided to insert another nasal gastric tube for liquid feeding. I still hated it, but I knew it would help Bill maintain his weight and nutrition levels.

A few days later, a resident suggested the possibility of implanting a feeding tube into Bill's stomach permanently. Then he could live on liquid feedings for the rest of his life.

"Bill enjoys cooking and eating and the social aspects that go with them," I said. "Life without such a simple pleasure would be of poor quality — no life at all, really."

The whole discussion left me wondering why this resident had already concluded Bill would never be able to eat on his own again.

16

NO OTHER OPTIONS

A WEEK LATER JUDY called to tell me that Bill's brothers wanted to visit.

"At least one of them will need to bring a wife," I said, only half joking. "I don't have the energy or time to think about meals or housekeeping, but otherwise we'll be glad to see them."

Judy, who was always willing to do her utmost, decided to travel with the three, each from a different town in the Maritimes, to make the visit and the drive easier on them, and on me.

It wasn't a very good time to see Bill, as I had warned them. I don't think he opened his eyes even once during their visits. A few days later, when they had to head for home, I knew they left believing they had said their last goodbyes. I found this so sad, because in my heart and soul I believed Bill would bounce back again.

The whole recovery process at the hospital took eight weeks from start to finish, from early September to the end of October.

Dr. Ellis ordered tight white support stockings for Bill to help with the clots; these were to be put on every morning and taken off every evening to keep the swelling down. I learned to roll them down as if I were putting them on myself. Baby powder shaken into them made them easier to put on. But still not easy. I struggled to get one unrolled and pulled all the way up Bill's leg, which was very puffy. I was huffing and puffing and swearing by the end of the first one. The second one was even worse.

Every nurse had her own ideas of how long the stockings should be left on, and even whether they were necessary. Eight hours? Twelve hours? Twenty-four hours? At the same time, Bill's ability to function changed dramatically and frequently: his body's pattern under duress. Even talking was a huge effort for him on some days.

Late one evening, near the end of October, as I just got home from the hospital, I received an unexpected call. It was Dr. Peter Carlson, the neuropsychologist of the Regional Community Brain Injury Services office in Kingston. Wendy, from the RCBIS office in Belleville, had told him I was terribly distressed and very fearful Bill was losing ground again. He asked if we could meet at his office. I needed some new input, and gratefully accepted his offer.

When we met, I was immediately struck by his expression, which seemed perplexed. I spent nearly an hour sharing my perceptions of the way Bill was being dealt with by the health care system.

"Everyone except Dr. Ellis and the oncologist acts as though they think he is about to die. No one seems to think that anything Bill has accomplished in the last six months means anything. He has no options for rehabilitation except me. It feels like nearly the whole system has deemed him disposable. Not worth trying to fix!"

I didn't let him get a word in edgewise.

"The agencies keep sending nurses who treat him like he is dying and support workers who aren't able to do what he needs, and most of them talk to me like I'm a lunatic and to him like he's on death's door! Don't these so-called professionals understand the oncology reports? 'No sign of residual malignant disease' is pretty clear, isn't it? I can't seem to get through to them that he isn't a terminally ill patient!"

I reiterated how angry I was that the regional hospital's team had given up on Bill so quickly.

Dr. Carlson tried to be sympathetic about my degree of discouragement but was guarded with his own opinions. However, understanding that Bill had already proved he had real potential, and that I was determined to advocate for him, he assured me his office would support me in developing a plan when Bill was more stable.

"It may be that what Bill needs might not be available from our agency, but we will provide support and advocacy and attempt to secure the help he needs," he said. "I will look into options, maybe find out about other programs."

ONE MORNING DR. ELLIS mentioned he'd arranged for the help of a new seizure disorder specialist on staff whom he considered one of the brightest and the best. As he had indicated, Dr. Allison Spiller was very knowledgeable, and very direct. She intended to look into Bill's specifics over the next while.

The last few days of October moved slowly, leaving me time to feel sad and lost. And to berate myself for what I saw as many mistakes I'd made. Bill still had the feeding tube in and was undergoing in/out catheters every eight hours. I mentioned to the nurse of the day that I was feeling overwhelmed and discouraged. She seemed to think I needed an update.

"The clots haven't diminished at all yet," she said. "Did they tell you that the tumour has regrown?"

It was a punch in the stomach.

"Why didn't the doctors tell me that?" I said when I was able to speak.

I cried and fretted outside Bill's room for ages until I met the neurosurgery resident, Trevor, and repeated the conversation.

"I hate it when this happens," he said with authority. "The nurse was wrong. Absolutely wrong. She gave you incorrect information."

Another valuable lesson for me: to consider the source before accepting information.

Finally the feeding tube was taken out, and Bill was eased back onto real food. Another step forward. But just as I got settled in at work a few days later, I received a call from the same young resident.

"Bill is okay," he quickly said. "But there's been an incident, and Dr. Ellis insisted I call you. The nurse helping Bill with breakfast was giving him orange juice off the tray when Dr. Ellis happened in. He was livid and demanded of the nurse, 'Didn't you know Bill is allergic to fruit?'"

Trevor told me Bill had been whisked to the critical care unit and the anti-allergic treatment had been administered.

"Bill is absolutely fine, no real harm done."

I shared my experience with Dr. Ellis a few days later.

"It's a perpetual problem," I told him. "My endless trips to the kitchen have resolved nothing. The trays still come with fruit on them. The big red sign over his bed that says he is allergic to fruits doesn't help. No one seems to see it. Including the people who are there to help him with meals. The people who are supposed to prevent harm."

The irony of it almost amused me. The brain surgeon knew Bill was allergic to fruit. The nurses whose care he was in every day of the week didn't.

With a going-home plan in the works, Dr. Ellis decided Bill should stay on the in/out catheters for a while, in the hope of stopping the recurring urinary tract infections.

"You can do it at home yourself," he said.

"No, I can't!"

"Yes, you can, and I will get the nurses to teach you. You *can* do this."

He sounded pretty confident. Certainly more confident than I felt.

"Well, I will try, but I am petrified."

What the charming doctor left out of his pep talk were the details: inserting the long tube into the penis and pushing it down until it enters the bladder, thus starting the draining. Oh Lord! People like me are the reason for the adage. "A little knowledge is a dangerous thing." I understood enough about blood thinners to know that a nick with a catheter tube could cause an internal bleed.

But I trusted the doctor's opinion and tried to talk myself into it. "Okay, Cath, this isn't brain surgery, and better you than yet another group of strangers poking and prodding him."

November 1 was the day Bill would leave the hospital. Again. Armed with the stockings, the catheter education, and my new fears, we prepared for our escape. Linda, the Community Care Access Centre liaison in the hospital, brought bags and bags of supplies we would need over the weekend.

"I will see to it that everything you need is at your house on Monday," she said. "If you need anything before that, call."

I appreciated her thoroughness. Her considerable optimism and endless encouragement gave my confidence a lift.

Dr. Ellis came in Saturday morning, on his day off, to say goodbye to Bill (and possibly "good riddance" to me). I had trouble articulating my gratitude for his help overseeing Bill this time, and then added, "Nothing personal, but even as I am very grateful, I never want to come back here again."

"Well, plan on it," he said.

There was something in how he said this that disturbed me, but I put it away for the moment. For now, we were on the road home again. Together.

17

AN ALIEN IN A NEW REALM

WHERE THE HELL TO start? The task ahead of us — helping Bill regain the strength, skills, and stamina he had lost in the last two months — was daunting just to think about it.

Dinner that first night, back in our own home, was a treasure. Sitting at the dinner table by the patio doors, Bill looked at his plate but didn't pick up his fork. Initiation was one of the brain issues he struggled with. I handed him the fork. The first piece he speared was a slice of potato. It skipped off the end of his fork, bounced onto the table, and bounced again, onto my plate. He followed its motion intently.

"Bull's-eye!" he said.

"Did you plan that, or was it just a lucky shot?"

"Just testing to see how your reflexes are. Not very good."

We took our time. Mainly because there wasn't any choice. Bill could not be rushed. We watched Jessie's antics and talked about the changes in the garden. Autumn, our favourite season, was on its way out, and we had missed most of it. I continued to put knife or fork in Bill's hand, just as a cue. I was relieved to see he was managing better than I had expected. I silently thanked Dr. Ellis for all the extra calories Bill had taken in through the feeding tube.

Inserting the in/out catheter that first night was a success, though my stomach lurched through the whole procedure. I was grateful when we could, once again, crawl into bed together.

The early-morning catheter and the stockings were now added to Bill's normal routine of getting into the shower chair, going into the bathroom, shaving, brushing his teeth, and the six other steps he followed to start his day. But those stockings! I sat on the bed on Bill's left and rolled down a stocking as if I were going to put it on my own leg. That would have been so much simpler. The damned things were tight enough to cut off the circulation in my hands.

"Okay, Hon, lift your left leg, please."

"Why?" he asked, as if we had never done this before.

"Because we need to get these stockings on your legs."

"Why?"

"Because they will keep the swelling down."

"What swelling?"

Bill obligingly lifted his leg. I started at his toes, trying to fit his foot into the tiny spandex sock part of the stocking first. I powdered the sock. I stretched it. It was like trying to get a bungee cord on his foot. Every time I got four toes in, one side would spring off. As I got that side in place, I would lose my grip on the other side. Finally, I got the whole foot in, which made it look like an overstuffed sausage. Then I unrolled the stocking up Bill's very long, very hairy leg.

Watching me struggle, Bill was quite amused. Once he had both stockings on, he hoisted one leg as high as he could and said, in his best Harpo Marx voice, "It would be easier to put a condom on a newel post."

He was right.

Inserting the catheter didn't go smoothly, either. As the bottle filled, I saw blood. Not pink. Not drops. Lots of deep red blood. I phoned the nursing agency and left my information. When the on-call nurse returned my call, she said, "It will be fine. It's not unusual. It's nothing to worry about."

How could I not worry? I was an alien in this new realm, without nursing training or skills, and this was a very invasive procedure — and I did understand the risks of the blood thinner Bill was taking. I could tell she just didn't want to trek out to our home. I begged her, imagining her with horns, tail, pitchfork, softening the picture when she agreed.

When she finally arrived, she was startled at the density of the blood. She stayed long enough to insert the next catheter herself. This time the fluid ran almost clear. Maybe it had been just a nick, but it was a frightening nick to me.

DURING EIGHT WEEKS in the hospital, Bill had lost some stamina and flexibility, although not as much as I had feared. And although it was discouraging to me, Bill was always willing to work through things. It was his willingness that refreshed my optimism and determination. We started at the beginning. Again. I heard my mother's voice many times, reminding me, "Count your blessings." I did.

Sitting side by side on the bed, we started working on getting him to sit up on his own again. Just a few minutes each session the first day. We added five-minute intervals each day, and in a week he was sitting independently for thirty minutes again. Sitting beside him on the bed I leaned sideways onto him, shoulder to shoulder. He pushed me back by leaning harder. Each time he pushed me sideways he laughed. The farther he could push me, the more he enjoyed it. This silly little game of ours was important. Balancing was something many brain-injured people could never do. It was very rewarding to see Bill improve each day.

Wendy from the RCBIS office in Belleville helped me set up a homemade pulley system she had seen. We rigged two rollers on the ceiling, shoulder width apart. A nylon cord ran through the rollers and down each side. By attaching a handle on each end and adjusting the length, we created a new exerciser.

Sitting on his shower chair (the very expensive tilting wheelchair was useless for this), Bill pulled one handle down beside the seat with his right hand. This pulled his left arm up into the air, giving it a good stretch. Then he pulled with his left arm. He did ten on each side, counting each out loud.

After three days of this new exercise he could do fifteen repetitions with each arm. By the end of the week he was doing twenty of each at each session — and pushing the ropes up, a much more difficult move. Counting helped him track his progress and increased his concentration. Most importantly, he was proud of his accomplishments.

In the middle of the second week, Linda, our Home Care case manager, called.

"I have great news," she said. "I've lined up a new physiotherapist for Bill. Her name is Cheryl. I need to tell you that she is a very new therapist, just out of school last year, but she has excellent references."

I had complained bitterly to Linda about the previous two therapists. Each had simply copied the reports and programs from the hospital physiotherapist. They offered nothing new, nothing hopeful. They may as well have shouted, "Bill is going to die anyway, so what do you want *me* to do?" Someone new, and hopefully less blasé, could only be an improvement.

Cheryl came to meet Bill and me on Saturday morning. She was very young, probably not more than twenty-four. At about five feet four, she had a tiny but athletic-looking body and very energetic body language. Shiny brown hair, big brown eyes, and an enthusiastic smile greeted me at the door. A solid, confident handshake told me she was ready for us.

She skirted around me and went to meet Bill, another good sign. Reaching out to shake hands, she introduced herself.

"Hi, Bill, I'm Cheryl. I'm your new physiotherapist. I'm really looking forward to getting to work with you."

Intrigued, he extended his hand, and the match was made.

Cheryl began her assessment, asking Bill to do various things — turn, roll, reach, lift a leg here, an arm there. She helped him sit up on the bed and poked, pushed, and watched some more. The puffiness in his face from the steroids, although greatly diminishing, still made him look like Humpty Dumpty to me, but Cheryl remarked it was normal and would not interfere with their mission. Most of her questions were aimed at Bill. She waited for his answers. This could take ten seconds, thirty seconds, or a minute or two. She waited.

At the end of the session, which had taken ninety minutes, she once again spoke directly to Bill.

"I think you and I will work very well together, Bill. I'd like to help you get back on your feet and get your independence back again. It will mean putting everything we've got into it, but I'm willing if you are. What do you think?"

"I'm in."

Their relationship was sealed.

I was mesmerized by the picture. Did Cheryl have different information than the two previous therapists? Or was she just not negative and jaded yet? Her enthusiasm made my soul sing.

Cheryl worked fiendishly with Bill. Her assessment was very different from the others. Her plan and approach was brand new, her own. She jumped over the old, standard routines, intent on getting Bill closer to doing things he deemed worthwhile. Their sessions always ran far beyond her "paid for" time. She never looked at her watch except to time something Bill was doing.

I watched from the landing. Cheryl climbed onto the bed, wiggling herself in behind Bill. "Lean way back into me, Bill. Great. Now sit up straight again." She positioned herself to grab him if he went too far forward, or fell backward. "Want to try transferring over to your chair without that lift contraption, Bill?"

"Affirmative."

The mechanical lift was not a favourite of Bill's. He said, "It makes me feel like I'm being delivered by the stork." Which was precisely how it looked.

Cheryl demonstrated for Bill. She placed a transfer board, thirty inches long, fourteen inches wide, well sanded and varnished to a smooth finish, on the bed under Bill's thigh, with the other end resting on the seat of the shower chair.

"Put your hands on the board, Bill."

She coached him to lift his butt and move it along the board a few inches. She performed a pantomime for him, showing him how to put more weight on his hands, arms, and legs. Patiently she repeated the steps over and over and over. Suddenly he was moving along the board. In one minute he was sitting on the chair.

Success!

"You are awesome, Bill!" Cheryl shouted, and they high-fived each other.

Bill was beaming. Cheryl was beaming. A solitary tear dripped down my cheek. These two were a perfect team.

Occasionally Cheryl included me in the workouts. Whenever she introduced something new, she showed both of us how to do it, supervising our first attempts, offering directions here, cautions there, and a whoop of excitement when we finally got it right. The basis for future success.

After their third or fourth session, when Cheryl had departed, I said to Bill, "You really like to work with Cheryl, don't you?"

"What's not to like?"

The perfect answer.

I WAS OFTEN frustrated, disheartened, and discouraged by the lack of interest and follow-through on the part of some of the nurses who worked shifts. Their work typically was strictly nursing, but Bill's needs were much more about rehabilitation than nursing, and when I asked them to help Bill with his exercises, I saw disbelief and that wife-in-denial look on many faces.

Bill's Home Care Book was growing. It now had a double-spaced front page:

Bill is not senile.
He is not hearing impaired.
He is not dying.
Please treat him accordingly.

Page 1. A list of his current medications; a reminder not to give him anything I had not prepared, because of his allergies; the protocol to follow if they had serious concerns. I was never unreachable, but just in case, call Dr. Mike Shirriff.

Page 2. The "daily intake and output" sheet: how much food Bill ate; how much he drank and what he drank; how much urine was extracted via the catheters; and the number of bowel movements. Maintaining a balance of calories, protein, liquids, and miscellaneous nutrients was vital. It was also difficult. This was a priority. Approaches and tips were detailed.

Page 3. The daily schedule. The entire day was spelled out from seven-thirty in the morning, detailing what Bill needed to do, and when. There were time slots for morning grooming, morning exercises, morning rest; time slots for cognitive activities, for lunch, an hour-and-a-half afternoon rest. Flexibility and strengthening activities took up most of the afternoon. There was time for scrapbooking or photo organizing, meant to be fun and engaging. The brain injury aspects, and the need to do things the same way repeatedly, were difficult to convey to new staff. I must have seemed incredibly anal-retentive to many.

When Cheryl joined Bill's team, we still endured a bevy of rotating shift nurses, but two personal support workers were becoming regulars.

Nancy, a quiet, slow personality, was still on the schedule. She was more accustomed to working with the elderly, whose primary needs seemed to be bathing and light housekeeping and someone to chat with them and make them feel important. Because she had seemed intimidated when I explained our regimen, I settled for knowing she would, at the very least, keep him safe for a few hours once a week.

Laurie was the opposite, a beacon of hope. She was enthusiastic and encouraging with Bill. Her blonde hair swung and bounced as she did many of his exercises alongside him. She was cute and young and vibrant, with a deep, bellowing laugh. In her he had a friend, not just a home care worker. She was helping him enjoy life.

"What did you and Laurie do tonight?" I often asked when I returned from work.

"We played darts," Bill was happy to report. "She's pretty good, but I won. We watched *Jeopardy*. I won."

I knew it was true. Laurie never let him win falsely. Over time they were usually even in the win-lose stats. I was grateful that it was always *Jeopardy* they watched, the only program ever on his schedule. So many times, with others, I had come home to discover the TV on an unusual channel. It infuriated me because watching *Dr. Phil*, *Oprah*, and soap operas was not part of their job.

"I love learning about Bill," Laurie said once. "Getting him to talk and to follow through on things is a real challenge, but it's really satisfying. Could we try a few different games, maybe a few on the whiteboard?"

This was the approach I had been pleading for. My husband had many limitations. To help him, a person needed to be able to see his potential and find ways to expand his world to help him develop.

Theresa, the nurse, still came weekly to assess Bill. She always treated Bill with dignity, respect, and humour; never like a child or invalid. With each visit she became more knowledgeable about him and continued to offer me tips and information. Bill was very comfortable with her. I trusted her completely.

Bill had opened up to Cheryl, Laurie, and Wendy because he saw them frequently. I continued pleading with the agencies to find shift nurses who could work consistently with Bill and be part of this team.

Wendy continued her work with Bill to help him cope with and reduce the brain issues he endured. Her years of experience and skill as a counsellor in the brain injury realm were invaluable. She was a physically imposing woman at six feet tall and had curly brown hair and big smile. She was a valuable resource in his day-to-day life, and he was more open with her than with most people. Sometimes I sat on the stairs, out of Bill's line of sight, and listened to their banter.

"Hey there, Bill, how are you today?"

"Tired and hungry."

"Didn't that wife of yours get you lunch today?"

"No, you can't get good help any more."

"Do you feel like you are making progress, Bill? Do you ever get days when you want to quit? Still willing to do these crappy exercises?"

Most often Bill offered positive, short answers. If he didn't answer, she rephrased her question, making it shorter, more direct. One goal she pursued was getting Bill to speak more. We hoped he eventually would initiate more conversations.

Wendy often tried to arrive for lunch. Meals were still my nemesis. Sometimes I made egg salad sandwiches. Thankfully, this was a favourite of both of them, because it was the high end of my skills. Munching away together — Bill ever so slowly — their conversation continued.

"Do you like your sandwich, Bill?"

"It's okay, but it's not lobster."

"Are you happy to be settled at home again?"

"Oh, for sure."

Wendy could carry on this process for an hour, between suggesting he eat more, or drink more, or swallow faster. She always waited until he answered her question. Wait, wait, wait. I asked if she could teach that skill to everyone. It irritated me when someone asked Bill a question, then immediately answered it for him. Most just didn't know that the time lapse between hearing, processing, and responding was significantly longer with most acquired brain injury patients.

18

YES, VIRGINIA...

In late november we gained two volunteer visitors. Linda, our Home Care case manager, had given Bill's name to Hospice in the summer. Bonnie, the coordinator, had visited in August and chatted amiably with us on our deck, enjoying the late flowers and cooler temperatures with us. She told us about the volunteers and how they gave their time to many people. (She never mentioned the word "palliative." I'm glad I didn't know they normally visited end-of-life people; if I had known, I would have declined.)

Before she could get us into their system, though, Bill had returned to the hospital.

As soon as Bill was back home, though, Bonnie arranged a visit from a man named Kevin MacDonald. He was willing to come and spend a couple of hours with Bill every Tuesday night. I was certain this new face would be a real bonus for Bill. I was always sad there were so few men in his day-to-day life. Earl and my brothers visited when they could, but it wasn't possible very often. Kevin's visits would be strictly social; he wasn't coming as a therapist or support worker or nurse.

I prepared Bill for Kevin's first visit, although he didn't understand why someone he didn't know was coming to see him.

Kevin was younger than I expected. He had an open, warm smile and a handshake to match. He was in the military, so he and Bill had a common denominator. The first night we just made small talk. Mostly Kevin and I. I took a picture of Kevin, and one of Kevin with Bill, for our album. Bill listened but didn't interject very much, even appearing to doze off at times.

During their first visits, Kevin did all the talking while Bill steadfastly ignored him. This visitor was not deterred, though. One evening, as I listened from the landing, I began to understand the unique gift Kevin brought. He had no expectations. He wasn't waiting for the *old* Bill MacLeod to surface the way, deep down, the rest of us were.

The second visitor, Pat, was a kind, sweet woman who brought knitting with her. I had arranged for her to visit during Bill's afternoon rest periods. This was time for me to grocery shop and take care of mundane errands. It also meant Bill didn't have to adjust to another stranger. During the several weeks she came I didn't realize she thought he spent virtually twenty-four hours a day sleeping. When I commented on how well he was progressing, she looked askance at me but was too polite to ask if I was insane. Later I showed her a video of Bill doing his daily exercise routines. She was stunned to see how much he could do. It was only then that I found out that being a hospice visitor usually meant visiting the dying. I asked that she not come back.

DECEMBER 2003 WAS upon us, and we stuck to our tradition of decorating the house and the tree early. Bill had the task of hanging the glass ornaments wherever he could reach. He leaned forward precariously in his chair, stretching toward the tree. He now had the muscle strength to pull himself back to an upright position, at least mostly. That is, he had progressed to knowing he *should* pull himself back up! He voiced opinions as to where things should be hung. It was a marvellous activity for us, just like old times. Kind of.

Another of his tasks was to remind Jessie that the tree was *not* to be peed on. Every time Bill picked up a globe, she leaped onto his lap and sniffed it, and Bill scratched her ears. Then she lost interest and jumped back down.

"Silly, silly dog," Bill always said, as he picked up another globe and the two of them went through the same routine.

What a pair. It was a joy to watch them. Listening to Christmas music playing quietly, looking at the tree and the decorations hanging on the fireplace often drew a sigh of contentment out of me. Happy Christmas season to us.

EARLY IN DECEMBER I called Dr. Shirriff's secretary. I always knew I could trust Laura to relay a message accurately. A home care nurse (another stranger) was very concerned about the sound of Bill's breathing. She felt strongly that he should be on an antibiotic. I did not agree, knowing that a severe bout of pneumonia years earlier had left Bill with a slight wheeze in his lungs, which often concerned nurses. But since I wasn't a doctor, I felt we needed a second opinion. I asked Laura to ask the doctor what he thought.

She called back and said, "Dr. Shirriff said he will drop by after work and check on Bill himself."

I was surprised and extremely grateful.

When the doctor arrived he got right to the task at hand, listening to Bill's chest and declaring him fine. Then he lingered, listening to the Christmas hymn playing on the stereo and looking at our fully decorated home. His "you won't be able to do this" look was gradually replaced with a sparkling, wide-eyed "you *are* doing this" look. Both his house call and his reaction: priceless.

THE MORNING OF Christmas Eve Bill and I talked about sending an e-mail to Dr. Ellis. The good doctor had given Bill his e-mail address when he learned at a follow-up appointment earlier in the month that Bill had a new computer. A friend had sent us an electronic greeting card that featured an outdoor winter scene complete with a brightly-lit tree. We agreed that Bill would forward it along with his best wishes. This actually was Bill's first time using the computer, which we had bought just before his surgery. It was intended to be a hobby for him while he recuperated.

In his wheelchair, with me at his right elbow, he decided what he wanted to say in his greeting. I printed the words on paper, in red ink, so he could refer to them. He searched the keyboard, one letter at a time. As he found each one he would thump down hard. With authority. At times he got distracted by all the other keys on the board. I silently asked Santa to help him get this right. He read various keys, asked, "What's that for? What does Shift mean? How do you say 'PgDn'?" and readily accepted my answer: "I haven't a clue."

After twenty-five minutes (which felt like one hundred and twenty-five to me) he had typed his very first e-mail: "Hi, Doctor Ellis. I am doing great. Hope you have a good Christmas. Bill MacLeod." He was excited to know it would go instantly to his favourite doctor. He did it! We high-fived each other with gusto.

After such success he wanted to send the card to his friends Earl and Ted. I groaned inwardly. This was torture for me. We went through the whole process again, and then again. Once the greetings were sent, though, I cherished the satisfaction in his smile.

At four-thirty an e-mail came in for Bill that read, "Glad you are doing well, Bill. Thank you for the neat card. Merry Christmas to you and your family. Peter Ellis."

Yes, Virginia, there is a Santa Claus…

OUR FORMER FAMILY room was now easily converted to a dining room. Our makeshift, multipurpose table looked as festive as every other year. Brenda shared Christmas dinner with us, and Al and Brenda Lee joined us on Boxing Day. They were all so patient and gracious with Bill while he took forever to finish his meal. They included him in the conversation as they always had.

After dessert, Bill and Al played a game of miniature pool on a tiny replica table, a gift from Santa. I was so glad not to be talking about brain injury or our current struggles.

This — the Christmas Bill was supposed to have spent in a nursing home — was a very, very special celebration.

PART THREE

*A LITTLE LESS
DRAMA, PLEASE*

19

THE NAG IN HIS LIFE

THE NEW YEAR ROLLED in with the shocking reminder it had been eleven months and one day since Bill's surgery. I sincerely hoped 2004 would be less dramatic.

As Kevin's weekly visits continued, Bill opened up to him more and more. Each Tuesday morning I would put Kevin's picture and the time he would visit on the whiteboard. The fourth time, Bill looked at the picture, read the name, and said, "Yeah. Kevin. He's a good guy."

Music to my ears.

I tried to stay out of the room during "their time." From upstairs I usually heard Cape Breton fiddle music coming from the CD player, although often they switched over to Floyd Cramer's piano renditions.

Bill owned a huge ball for exercising. One evening Kevin produced it and they began a game of their own. I could hear bouncing, a pause, another bounce, a pause, and yet another bounce and a pause. I reckoned the visitor wasn't running back and forth playing both sides of this game. Bill must be participating. Wow!

It wasn't long before Kevin had learned about Bill's skills and his personality. In the midst of a game, Bill would suddenly catch the ball and hold onto it. He would examine it all around. What was he looking for? Nothing. He was patiently waiting for his guest to be distracted. Then, quick as a flash, he would fire it at his victim, catching him off guard. Bill would smirk, and then chuckle.

This was great hand–eye coordination work. It was great reflex work. It was just plain fun for Bill.

In just a few short weeks I had developed a trust in Kevin that was rare for me. I knew I could leave them on their own and that Kevin would call if he needed me and would keep Bill engaged. He was no longer a volunteer visitor. He was *our friend* Kevin. And he was very special.

THE NEW YEAR brought new advances, new goals, and new challenges. Cheryl worked doggedly with Bill, adding new building blocks to his progress each week. She encouraged and prodded him to put more and more weight through his legs and into his feet. I often watched, unnoticed, from the stairwell.

Sitting beside him on the bed, reminding him about his posture, Cheryl leaned her upper body way out, feet firmly planted, arms reaching. Bill did the same. She leaned way back, resting her head on the pillows. Bill did the same. She reached her arms up high and raised herself up to sitting. Bill…well, Bill gave it his best effort. They laughed long and loud. She offered her elbow for enough support to right him. Bill said thanks, but in a tone that implied he didn't really need her help.

Each week Cheryl worked diligently to guide Bill through the transfer process, cueing him and lugging him when necessary to get him from bed to chair. Being small was no hindrance to her; she was feisty, energetic, and optimistic. A very good influence and a constant reminder to me I could do much of this work between their sessions.

Sometimes she introduced new activities to use a different muscle group. Just for fun. All these things were improving Bill's coordination and balance, and his spirit. Occasionally I was invited to join them. Cheryl took me through ways to do specific things, emphasizing how to keep him safe. This very helpful information enabled us to branch out into other areas on our own. "Our Cheryl" was the physiotherapist of our dreams.

Posture was an ongoing struggle, but Laurie was gifted at getting Bill to sit up tall, reach for things, look up at the television perched on the top of the wall unit (Wendy's idea). Bill was making real progress with her.

ON FEBRUARY 14, when I got back from work, there was a package and an envelope on our table. A note attached to the envelope read, "Do not open this until after the card and parcel." Inside the beautiful card was a handwritten message: "Happy Valentine's Day. I Love You. H. W. MacLeod," signed with Bill's very distinct signature. The package contained a lovely clear glass jar full of red and white jellybeans. In her note Laurie had written,

> *Catherine, Bill single-handedly put every jellybean in the jar for you, except the ones he ate! He told me what he wanted to write in the card, but when he tried to write, he became fidgety and frustrated, so he let me write it for him. However, he did "significate" the I Love You, signed his name, and helped me wrap.*
>
> *Happy Valentine's to you both.*
> *Laurie*

This was a very special gift from Bill, and a treasured one from Laurie. I was overcome with gratitude to her for helping Bill achieve a sense of accomplishment in this and many other things.

She always encouraged his participation and helped him discover new (old) things he could do again.

Unfortunately, a disagreement that she had with her agency caused her to quit just a few weeks later. We lost someone valuable, and it was some time before we found another PSW with similar skills and traits. It was a sad event for Bill. For both of us.

IN EARLY MARCH, Bill reminded me that his sister Verna's birthday was approaching. Bill had five sisters, so there always seemed to be another birthday around the corner. Still, I would not have remembered. I bought a card and watched as Bill signed "Harold W. MacLeod." I put my own note in the card, telling Verna about Bill remembering her special day. She had come, with Judy, to see him right after his surgery but hadn't been able to return again. This was his very special gift to her.

We did another card in April for Kevin's birthday, this signed with Bill's more formal signature, "H. W. MacLeod." I made copies of all these cards, to have forever. Treasures in the memory box.

In mid-January we had started doing floor exercises on our own. I used the mechanical lift to lower Bill onto an exercise mat. He understood this was to make his legs strong enough to get back to standing and walking. He put his heart and soul into it. Once he was on the floor, I asked him to roll to the right and stretch his left arm and hand toward the wall unit. Then I asked him to do it in the other direction. He struggled to accomplish this. Leg lifts, which progressed from a few inches off the ground to thirty inches, got to be much easier.

This all occurred in just a few weeks. Lying on his back he bench-pressed a variety of articles: a broom stick, a hockey stick, a broom stick with a weight on it, and as many other accessories as we could dream up. We had become masters of improvisation.

I had learned about the value of video the year before at the Acquired Brain Injury conference and when I was able to get a video camera I began taping our "sessions." By making a tape of his workout, I hoped one day Bill soon would be able to follow it on his own.

When I played it back as a complete workout, though, I was shocked and deeply saddened. Even as I watched his remarkable progress, I hurt for both of us.

Suddenly I saw myself as I imagined Bill saw me. I was the nag in his life now.

This had never been true in our former life. Yet there I was. "Do this, do that, do it again, turn there, twist here, stretch more, roll again, no not like that." Most of the time he accepted all of this good-naturedly, but occasionally his eyes flashed and he snapped, "For God's sake, Cath, I am not five years old." His rebuke was an equalizer.

I thought about all the indignities that were now imposed on Bill. By me. The person I loved more than I could even describe was forced to have me assist him with the most intimate acts of daily living, from helping him wipe his bum to helping him cut his food. I prayed to the universe that I truly was doing the right thing for him, which at least helped me shrug off the despair and move onward again.

THE NEXT PHASE of our workout was scarier. Bill lay on his back on the floor and raised his legs into the air. I leaned my body onto his feet. He bent his knees slowly toward his chest, and then he straightened his legs up again with my full weight on his feet.

The little devil on my shoulder hissed, "This is what early, proper rehab could have done. And a whole lot sooner."

It took two weeks, working five days a week, to get to this point. We repeated the same process with his arms. He raised and lowered me right above himself, our hands and our prayers entwined. This brought forth some private jokes, another reminder the old Bill was still in there! These were amazing rides for me, and I captured them on video, too. I made copies and sent them to his family on the coast, keeping several for us, for show-and-tell.

Viewing the tape launched Cheryl into deciding it was time for Bill to *stand*. She walked Bill and me through every motion of this very scary process. Not much taller than I, she was confident that both of us could do this with Bill. She got us started. I tried to get confident. Bill used the electric buttons on the long cord to raise the bed to its maximum. He wrapped his arms around me, and I wrapped mine around him. We loved that part! He worked to put all his weight down into his legs and feet and hoist his fanny up off the bed and into my body.

Day after day we worked, gaining maybe an extra inch or two off the bed each time. Wendy often helped with this part. As I stood in front of Bill, she stood behind me, very near at hand. I hoped that, since she was nearly as tall as Bill, she would catch us both if we started to fall. Fortunately, that was never tested.

Wendy could see the muscles in his legs working. Weight bearing was well underway. He got better at keeping those feet planted firmly on the floor and leaning forward at the same time.

One day as we went through the usual routine, something unfamiliar happened. Suddenly I felt something different. Bill's weight had transferred completely from me to his own legs. Oh, my God! *This was my miracle.* For all intents and purposes, he was standing! He was grinning. Wendy and I were whooping and crying and high-fiving him.

By the middle of April Bill stood twice, for thirty seconds each time, without any support from me. No stopping us now!

I recalled the first physiotherapist at our local hospital, and her declaration: "He'll never be able to sit up or stand on his own." Perhaps I would send her a picture of this Kodak moment.

KEVIN WAS STILL building his unique relationship with Bill. They preferred to be left alone. They played air hockey. They played darts. They enjoyed their time. For the first time since this journey began, I could take a book, a fun book, to our former bedroom upstairs and unwind.

Kevin was proficient at getting Bill to eat and drink. He understood the problems Bill had experienced as a result of dehydration and not enough calories. He was diligent, reminding him, "Take a bite," or, "Have a drink of your shake."

As opponents, they continued to throw around different sizes of balls. Kevin was amazed at Bill's reflexes, and his sneakiness. I heard them using the pulleys, challenging each other, followed by uproarious laughter. Whatever their jokes, they did not usually share them with me. This was guy stuff.

Often Kevin lamented at the end of their visit, "He beat the crap out of me at air hockey again!"

To which Bill laughed and added, "Well, he's really not very good."

These were the sounds of a very happy Bill.

Not all visits were a success, though. Sometimes Bill retreated, going who knew where. Sometimes it was because of fatigue. Other times it may have been the result of overstimulation during the day. Kevin was never deterred. He waited patiently, and waited some more. He knew instinctively not to answer his own question. If Bill didn't, or couldn't, or wouldn't answer, Kevin left it there rather than fill in his own response. Because of their common connection to the Air Force, Kevin sometimes, in desperation, did a complete military monologue, hoping to engage Bill. Eventually, though, he started to bribe Bill. I never knew what he was willing to trade for a single word!

CHERYL AND WENDY continued to brainstorm with me. Cheryl described new piece of equipment, a Standing Frame, and said she could get one on trial. The contraption was a seat, a front and back brace, and a hydraulic system. By using a lever, Bill could push himself from sitting to an upright position, securely encased so there was no risk he would fall. Doing this every day could help him build the strength and stamina and balance to become much more independent. It was designed for paraplegics to enable them to roll around at home and work and pursue their jobs and lives. It offered great potential.

It also was six thousand dollars. There was no way I could come up with that much money. My credit card was maxed out, I had cashed in our GICs already, and I still wasn't back to work full-time. Here was part of the fix, and I couldn't get it for him.

With encouragement from these two inventive women, we developed another idea. I asked Bill's friend Duane to acquire a parachute harness. With his, Wendy's, and Cheryl's help, we got Bill into the harness, and, voilà, we airlifted him with the mechanical lift. At first he was apprehensive, still not fully grasping that he couldn't just stand up on his own. But once up in this bizarre rig, he could straighten to his full height, stand on both feet, and march on the spot, with a very different view of his surroundings from up there. An exciting experience for all of us.

I HAD NEVER, ever shared anyone's negative pronouncements with Bill, nor did I ever intend to. He was completely informed by Dr. Ellis and Dr. Madernos of the surgery results and the pathology and the concerns that might arise. What he would or wouldn't be able to do, in someone else's opinion, I kept to myself. He was unique, and *they* didn't know his determination. They also didn't know the strength of our commitment. Nor of our creativity.

20

D-DAY

FOR MONTHS WENDY, FROM the RCBIS office in Belleville, had been pushing me to request a specific personal support worker from the agency, and I had. Several times. No luck. Jan had worked for the Brain Injury Services office in Kingston before moving to our area. She had considerable training, skill, and background in brain injury rehabilitation. But because no positions for her specific skills in this community were available, she was working as a personal support worker, mainly with seniors, mainly doing housework for them. What an incredible waste.

Was I asking too nicely? I nudged my attitude up a little. (A lot!) In three days I was told Jan was coming to meet us. I was relieved, but irritated at the same time. I had pleaded with the agencies to send people with her skills from day one. Why hadn't they sent her long before this? Didn't they know her background?

As she introduced herself with a very firm, confident handshake,

I knew she was the right one. Jan sported a casual, simple haircut, no makeup. She dressed simply, neatly. She was bright and enthusiastic and understood some of my frustrations. Immediately she went to Bill and struck up a conversation. Her experience with others with similar cognitive deficits was encouraging. She was interested in our agenda, and was optimistic, open-minded, and truly wanted to make a difference.

Even after reading *Bill's Home Care Book*, she was still interested.

I warned her about me, too, and how concerned and intense I could be, and she was still interested.

She scrutinized his photo album and videos and saw I wasn't exaggerating his progress. Based on her practical comments and interactions with Bill, I knew in my gut she was going to be good for him. And for me. I liked her direct approach. Most importantly, Bill liked her.

Jan joined his harem the following Thursday, working two evenings one week, one the next week. It felt so good to leave him in the hands of someone smart and keen. What a difference. I couldn't imagine I would ever be calling the case manager to complain about this girl. (I never did.)

MY CONCERNS ABOUT the financial issues surrounding our home program were growing like a monster, though. I had had no idea how costly everything about this process would be, and sometimes the worry affected my interaction with others. I worked hard to keep most difficult issues from Bill. He had enough to cope with. But so often I ached for the time when I would have honestly shared my concerns with the man who had always been my compass and anchor.

Jan, Bill, and I communicated easily, smoothly. Training was so much easier, and faster, than it had been with the others. I had been exhausted after every session with someone new and then had lain awake at night trying to remember if I had missed anything. I had resented the training of so many workers because it devoured enormous amounts of time and energy; time and energy I wanted and needed to spend with Bill accomplishing things and being husband and wife.

Wendy told me about a piece of equipment used in a number of rehab centres: the Ex N' Flex, an electronic pedalling machine, perfect for someone in a wheelchair. Once the feet are strapped in, the user can pedal forward or backward by increasing and decreasing pressure.

As soon as it arrived it became a mainstay of Bill's daily workout. He started with a five-minute session, twice a day, but every few days, as his stamina and leg strength improved, we increased the sessions by five-minute increments. Part of his workout included keeping track of how long he pedalled forward, and switching to the reverse every five minutes. In just a few weeks he was doing two half-hour sessions every day. It was a great exercise both physically and cognitively.

UNDERSTANDING HOW LIMITED Bill's world had become, Cheryl was working toward helping him do transfers in and out of the car. We set a date and called it D-Day. This would require strategic planning, but Cheryl was ready. I was apprehensive. I desperately wanted him to be able to do this, but what if he got hurt? What if Cheryl got hurt?

On that lovely, sunny morning in early April, we got all the equipment ready. The vastly expensive wheelchair was quite useless for this endeavour, too. Cheryl and Bill were using his shower chair, with its flip-up arms and the transfer board under him bridging the gap to the seat of the car. I watched in awe. She directed Bill step by step, even lifting him by the seat of his pants to help him shuffle over. Getting his long legs and big feet into a low-slung, two-seat car was awkward.

Suddenly I realized, "Oh, my God, he is in our car!" I raced inside for the camera and the dog. Bill looked totally underwhelmed, as if he had been in the car just yesterday.

Cheryl beamed from ear to ear, saying, "We did it, Bill," as she high-fived him. Another Kodak moment.

I wanted to make good use of this feat.

"Where would you like to go for a drive, Hon?"

"Tim Hortons."

After ordering at the drive-through, we drove, drinks and cookies in hand, the few miles to Kevin's house to share this momentous event, with the CD playing "On the Road Again," the window down, and the puppy likely thinking we had gone quite mad.

We reversed the procedure to exit the car when we got home. It wasn't with Cheryl's finesse, but we managed. Together. We did it again the next day, in and out, just the two of us. Not smooth yet, but mission accomplished. The third time, though, was nearly a disaster. The board slipped, Bill ended up sitting on the very edge of the floor panel, and I was in a frenzy.

"Well, what do we do now, Einstein?" my darling asked, winking.

We got sorted out eventually, and I learned more valuable safety tips. Now we needed a wheelchair that would fold up if this success were to truly benefit Bill. It would increase Bill's independence in a host of areas. Financing a two-thousand-dollar wheelchair at a hundred dollars a month was easier than I expected.

I was still battling the little demon in my mind that kept tempting me to throttle the hospital physiotherapist for her closed mind.

LATER I LEARNED about "change-of-function status." The Ministry of Health funds mobility devices based on a patient's current status through its Assistive Devices Program. If that status improves or declines, it funds a more suitable piece of equipment — but you have to have a therapist sign off on it. If I had known about this, I could have applied for the lighter, easier, and more versatile chair. But it was too late: we had already shelled out another couple of thousand dollars on this one.

But now, finally, we could go wherever we wanted. Bill could rejoin his community. No stopping us now.

21

UNEXPLAINED ABSENCES

FOUR DAYS LATER A grey, drizzling spring rain was falling. It was a perfect day for lolling around doing small stuff. The fireplace took the chill out of the air and added to the cozy mood. I heaped an armful of warm clothes, fresh from the dryer, onto Bill's lap as he sat in his wheelchair. Laughing and taking a deep sniff of the fresh-scented clothes, he pushed everything onto the bed. Folding his clothes was a task he enjoyed. Spotting a royal blue golf shirt, he pulled it from mid-pile and shook it vigorously.

"This one wrinkles fast. I love this shirt. It's such a great colour."

Once he had it folded perfectly, the front smooth, both sleeves wrapped to the back, he set it aside. Next he rescued a pair of flannel pants from the heap. Shaking them out, he laid them over his knees and smoothed a crease into the legs, enjoying the feel of the soft fabric, and laying them carefully over a hanger. Bill loved his clothes, and always enjoyed the routine of choosing his outfit each morning.

Laundry dispensed with, I dusted and polished the furniture. Bill cleaned the full-length mirror that stood on the floor. A gift from his sister Verna, it was multipurpose. He sat in front of it in the morning to shave, brush his teeth, brush his hair, and fix his shirt collar. I would tilt it so he could watch his position as he did his floor exercises. The more he watched his reflection, the more he was able to self-correct his posture. This meant fewer things for me to nag about.

Cleaning it himself was another job he took pride in. Watching him turn it, spray it with Windex, and wipe it down with a paper towel, no stranger would guess he had any brain problems. He smiled when I mentioned what a great team we were. He still loved our life, and his contribution to it.

DINNER WAS BASED on what vegetables Bill wanted to peel. "Carrots, potatoes, and turnips today." We watched a golf tournament while he laboured over his meal preparations. It was a warm, familiar, and comforting feeling to be doing something so normal together. His progress was exciting. And now that we could go out in our own car, I was certain more advancements were coming for him.

I glanced at Bill to see his reaction to an amazing golf shot. He was staring. He stared for thirty seconds. Not a blink, not a sound. I saw him gulp, three or four times. Then an eye twitched. It looked like a wink. Suddenly, as if a switch had clicked, he was back, focused on the golf shot, commenting on the prowess of the player. Tiger Woods had regained the lead.

My peaceful mood started to crumble. Something was wrong.

Several hours later, settled in bed for the night, I watched it happen again. Bill was completely unaware he had been "absent."

The next day the "absence" seizures became more pronounced and more severe: A slight twitch of the right eye. Gulping, deep and rhythmic. Slowly, the right hand and arm reaching out into the air. Head turning to the left. Shoulders, torso following. Right knee bending to follow. A shiver. All in slow motion.

Then it was over. For me, though, another problem was just beginning.

Kevin came to visit in the evening, and despite Bill's condition he stayed to help.

"I can't believe how 'in tune' Bill and you are," he said. "What an incredible connection you have. How you can tell that something is going to happen before it does."

Kevin had plenty of questions, and his learning curve about seizures was intense and rapid.

"I didn't know before either that there are dozens of types of seizures, or that they present in so many different ways," I explained, as we watched and timed the durations of each spell.

Their frequency was increasing. At first only lasting thirty to forty seconds, by the next day they were lasting a minute and a half.

The local lab had home service for people unable to go to their office, as long as your doctor authorized it and you could pay for it. They came once, twice, sometimes three times a week to do blood work for Bill. When in doubt, I sent urine samples, too. The morning of day two I sent a sample. Most often an infection was at the root of these "partial seizure" episodes, so this might fast-track the answer.

My morning call to Dr. Shirriff was returned promptly. I shared the information, and the next day, Wednesday, he came to see things for himself. By then the seizures were both stronger and longer.

We agreed Bill should go to the hospital in Trenton; Dr. Shirriff, meanwhile, would contact Dr. Spiller, the seizure specialist in Kingston. Ambulance travel to the local hospital in Trenton was calm — no sirens needed this time. I chuckled, noting Bill and I were on a first-name basis with the paramedics. They asked the routine questions only because they were supposed to.

Once in the Trenton ER, more blood testing was done. Low hemoglobin. The ER doctor strongly suggested a transfusion. I was reluctant. Like most people, I hadn't forgotten our tainted-blood scandal.

"What would you be doing if this was your partner?" I asked him.

Without hesitation, he said, "I would be saying yes."

I finally agreed, and the transfusion was started. I prayed it was the right decision. Hours later, Bill was admitted to a room — thankfully, a private room.

Dr. Shirriff was very open to Dr. Spiller's advice. I so appreciated that he wasn't egotistical and arrogant like the specialists here at this small hospital who had supervised Bill's care last year. He adjusted the medications several times over several days, but it didn't stop the seizures. They were intensifying and becoming much more frequent.

And I was becoming more frantic. Fear was the devil I danced with most of the time. I sat beside Bill all day and through the night, hoping I could talk him through each seizure and monitor the times, duration, and the intensity of each one.

The night nurse, irritated by my constant presence, said, "You are just overanxious. We can take care of him, and we will. You don't need to stay. We do know what to do."

She was right about the first part. I was extremely anxious. Our history, and my distrust of this hospital, was something I still couldn't get past. Past events were etched in my memory. But I wanted her to understand my side of this picture.

"I'm not here to watch for mistakes. I'm not here to check up on you or the other staff. I'm not here to challenge any of you. I am here because I know what these seizures do to my husband and I don't want him to be alone when they happen. That's all."

By day four Dr. Shirriff and I agreed: Bill was significantly worse, slipping into those periods of "decline of consciousness" again. He needed to go to Kingston General Hospital. It was Saturday morning, but Dr. Shirriff decided to contact Dr. Spiller again. They conferred, exchanged information, and agreed that Bill needed her direct care. The seizures were taking a toll on him. I was relieved when Dr. Shirriff told me Dr. Spiller would make the arrangements to have Bill admitted to KGH that day.

As I packed Bill's things, and prepared him for another ambulance trip, I did my best to make this sound like good news. Between seizure bouts he was terribly fatigued, but still talking to me. Looking out the window at the rain and drizzle, he said, "God, I feel like shit."

At two o'clock Dr. Shirriff walked into Bill's room. It was pouring rain, and his day off. I realized he was not there to bring good news.

"Catherine, I hate to have to tell you this, but Bill won't be going to Kingston General today. Dr. Spiller is still new there and she didn't realize, until she tried to make the arrangements, that it isn't as simple as she expected. The hospital has policies and protocols."

"Are you saying that a seizure disorder neurologist, after consulting with the very well-informed family doctor, both believing that the patient should be in neurology care, cannot make that happen?" I heard the hysteria in my voice.

"Yes," was his simple response.

"What is the matter with that hospital? Do they not trust their own specialists to make these decisions? Does management know more about seizures and the potential risk than she does? Do they not realize what damage is happening while she gets a 'policy' lesson?"

I tried not to shout. This wasn't his fault, but I was seething and scared. Numerous more calls were exchanged between the doctors. They were as distressed as I. Sunday's update was the same: Bill still couldn't be transferred.

My words came out as if from an automatic weapon.

"What the hell are those administrative assholes thinking? Do they just not give a shit about Bill? Are they trying to keep this expense in Trenton? The next time you speak to the neurologist, please ask her to tell those bean counters that my very first call tomorrow morning will be to our lawyer! Isn't the regional hospital's mandate to provide care to its taxpayers who cannot get what they need in their local hospital? And clearly, you and Dr. Spiller and I agree that Bill needs neurology help."

Several hours later Dr. Shirriff called from his home, sounding very relieved. Bill would in fact be transferred to Kingston General that day. We speculated that Dr. Spiller may have passed on my comments about my lawyer to her bosses. I was anxious to leave before anyone could change their mind and fretted while waiting for the ambulance. Bill had been in dire straits here for several days, and for several days before that at home.

I swung between being Dr. Jekyll and Mrs. Hyde: trying to be calm and confident and soothing with Bill between seizure bouts, and, when Bill couldn't hear or see me, fussing and fuming at anyone who came within fifty feet of me. This whole scenario was a travesty. Our world was crashing around us again, and this blockade was about rules and protocol, not Bill's well-being. Again.

I had never realized or expected it would be so difficult and enraging to advocate for my husband.

Once the paramedics had Bill in their care, I calmed down a little. I tried to express to Dr. Shirriff how thankful I was to him for being so available, for advocating for Bill, and being tolerant of my ranting. I joked with Bill later about the change of heart Dr. Mike had undergone since Bill's early days in Complex Continuing Care. All the way from "not suitable for rehabilitation" to cheering Bill on as he improved.

"He's come a long way, Baby!" we said in unison.

COFFEE IN HAND, alone in the car, I followed the ambulance, musing about all the ups and downs Bill had been through. We had always tried not to live in fear. Expecting the best outcome for anything was our best defence, as that allowed us to be optimistic. Those attitudes were more valuable to me now than ever, but they were elusive at times. Today I felt as if I was living most of my time in the state of fear. I was not stoical. I was not strong. I was swamped by my fears, but I dared not share them with anyone.

I was worried now that even a hint of my state of mind would give others the opportunity to say, "I told you so," and that they might use it as another excuse for not helping Bill.

22

"THINGS JUST HAPPEN"

THE NEUROLOGIST ON ROTATION was the same one who had headed the team that deemed Bill "nursing-home disposable" the previous year. He was well respected, but I had a serious grudge against him, which made me even more grateful that Dr. Spiller would really be overseeing Bill this time. I knew she was the one who would make any changes in medication and testing and would come and talk to us personally and consult us first. I had full confidence in her, because, like Dr. Ellis, she didn't mince words. She was direct and straightforward with information but also compassionate, empathetic, and patient. Essential for anyone dealing with me now. I was confident Bill was safe in her care.

I stayed with Bill in the neuro critical care unit as much as possible. I had become fixated on the details of his care, no longer fully trusting the system here, either. I tried not to obsess over tracking his seizures by time and counting them, but to me, whether they improved or didn't would influence the next course of action.

Workdays were agonizing, and I was indebted to my sister and our friends for filling in some of the hours so he wasn't always with strangers. By now I was always afraid something else would happen to him when I wasn't with him. That no one would be there to talk him through the revolving events. They must be horribly painful and frightening. Would anyone remind him I was at work? That I'd be back? Would anyone comfort him and keep his spirits from sinking? Talk to him? Encourage him? My ad hoc education and neurosis about the health care system had entered a new chapter.

Dr. Spiller told me about a new anti-seizure medication. She was confident it would work well for Bill, and it was known to have far fewer side effects. But, of course, there was a hitch. She wasn't allowed to try it immediately. The new drug was not yet on the "approved-for-payment list" from the Ministry of Health. Before she could administer what she believed would work best, she first had to prove that she had tried all the drugs currently listed!

I could only wonder. Was this meant to be a cost-saving measure? A management "control" tool? My logic screamed: If Bill had to stay in the neuro critical care unit for days or weeks until she was allowed to try a potentially better drug, could that really be a money saver? Was there a dollar value put on the cost to Bill? And to me? Bureaucracy!

I still had the book *Where Is the Mango Princess?* by the American Cathy Crimmins who believed our system was so much better than that in the United States. I was no longer convinced. Day after day, as I watched my husband suffer dozens of these multiple-seizure episodes, that black hole of despair flirted with me constantly. I felt impotent. I couldn't help him. He couldn't help me.

Arriving at the hospital Friday evening in late April, after a very long work week and workday, I asked the nurse if she knew how many seizures Bill had that day.

"None," she said.

None? That was impossible, or at least highly improbable. I had a flashback to the nurse at Trenton who didn't know tremors from seizures. Sitting beside Bill's bed, my count began within a very few minutes.

When she came by the next time, I asked, "Do you know what these particular seizures look like? Because Bill has had several just in this last very short while. I'm not trying to give you a hard time, and I have great respect for the work you do, but if Dr. Spiller is told these have abated, much less stopped completely, she will think the current medication is working. Which, clearly, it is not."

The nurse assured me an exact count didn't matter.

"Maybe not, but there is a huge margin of error between zero seizures and twenty seizures in one eight-hour shift, which influences the course of treatment for Bill."

My tone was sharper than I intended, but I was already worrying about whether more brain cells were being affected while we waited for the approval to try the new drug.

The next morning, the new day nurse approached Bill's bed, holding a syringe full of the anti-seizure medication. As soon as I saw the colour of the mixture, a light purple, I knew it wasn't the right drug.

"Before you inject that, would you do me a favour, please?" I said. "I think that's either not the correct drug or it's the wrong dosage." I kept my tone soft, smooth, and non-combative.

Her response was none of those. "Of course it's the right one. I just got it from the trolley. You know, it's not helpful when you are here checking up on us. We really do know what we're doing."

"Well, first of all, I'm sorry if you think that's why I'm here. It is not. But, I also think it's possible even for professionals to goof now and then. All I am asking is for you to go back and double-check your information. I've seen this drug often enough to know that the one in your hand isn't the right one."

I was still managing to keep my tone even, but when she reached for the tube to inject the concoction I put aside all pretence of nice.

Reaching for her arm, I said, "You are not injecting that until you go back and double-check. If I'm wrong, I will buy your dinner."

She stomped away, picked up Bill's chart, and walked out of the room. She was gone for ten minutes. When she returned she carried a syringe of a pale green substance I recognized. Without a word she began administering the correct medication.

I tried to smooth over our conflict.

"Honestly, I am here to do whatever I can for Bill. If that means that sometimes I see a mistake, it certainly doesn't mean I think you're all stupid. Far from it. But there's a human error factor in everything, and sometimes things just happen."

She didn't respond.

FIVE DAYS AFTER Bill's admission to Kingston General and with no decline in his seizures, Sandra, a nurse who knew Bill well, pointed out that he was developing contractures. The muscles and ligaments in his legs were tightening up, preventing him from straightening his legs. Contractures. Another new problem. I knew just enough to realize this newest problem would very possibly prohibit Bill from straightening his legs enough to bear weight again. Shit.

Finally, when none of the other drugs had worked and Bill's time in Purgatory was served, Dr. Spiller was allowed to start him on the new — but not yet listed — drug. Within three days it proved highly effective. His seizures decreased, then totally subsided. In just a few days, his degree of consciousness had almost returned to his previous level, and he was moved to a regular room on the neuro floor.

I ALWAYS HAD our photo album close to hand like a much-loved Bible. I had started taking photos of Bill doing his daily activities while he was still at Trenton Hospital. I continued the practice at home, which included taking pictures of him doing each new activity with me and with visitors, therapists, and home care staff. It had also become known, to me at least, as the "screw you album," because it bristled with documentation I could brandish when anyone pigeonholed Bill as a hopeless case. I dreamed of one day showing it to the entire medical team that had recommended a nursing home.

One day during this time I saw the social worker in the hallway who had been on Bill's team the previous year. The team that had sentenced him to a nursing home. I invited her to Bill's room. Making very little effort to hide my resentment, I showed her Bill's photo album, depicting his home life. A picture really is worth a thousand words. She was speechless.

"Does anyone on the medical team who managed Bill's case have any idea what complex continuing care in our local hospital is like?"

"No, we don't have the time to get out to those places."

"Well, you all bloody well should before you choose that as a solution."

Even I was surprised by the intensity of my anger as I briefly described what that experience had been like for us.

"You need a lot more information about these places before sentencing anyone else to a geriatric warehouse."

She offered no response.

A FEW DAYS later, with the seizures now controlled, Bill was discharged. This time, two weeks after his admission to Kingston General, I was very anxious to get him out the hospital door. I was conflicted: grateful for the care and skill available here, yet angry beyond words at a system that allowed new problems to develop because of policies or saving money.

I couldn't help speculating. Would Bill have gone home much sooner without the delay for the new drug? Would he have spent much less time in the neuro critical care unit? Would the lengthy seizures that had led to his now painfully contracted legs have been avoided?

23

A PRIVATE CAVE

AND SO WE CROSSED the threshold of our home. Again. Seizure problem solved. Serious new problem gained. I had not truly grasped how severely the leg contracture problem would impede Bill's progress.

My first call was to Cheryl. I knew I could rely on her expertise, experience, and interest to guide us through this new issue, since the realm of contractures was totally foreign to me. Bill and I talked a lot about this new and painful leg problem, and from what I had learned, it was something that could be overcome with time, hard work, determination — and Cheryl's guidance. He was looking forward to exercising with her again.

When I called, though, I was surprised and saddened to learn she had accepted a full-time position at the local hospital. I understood her decision but still felt completely abandoned. "What next?" I moaned.

Once composed, I called Linda, Bill's Home Care case manager, who quickly said, "I'm working on getting a replacement therapist already."

When Paulo, the new physiotherapist, finally arrived, I introduced him to Bill. He did a brief, very basic assessment, and then proceeded to test Bill's legs for flex. There wasn't much. He pressed down on each leg, one at a time, applying enough pressure that Bill winced. His approach seemed excessively forceful, but I didn't want to get off on the wrong foot by voicing my thoughts. It was a very short visit, less than thirty-five minutes. But, of course, we were used to Cheryl, who had often stayed overtime to get something done.

The second visit, a week later, was much the same, and my concern about too much force was heightened. He explained several different exercises to Bill and demonstrated them. I noticed him looking at the clock several times. Was he late for something more important? As the therapist went out the door, Bill commented, "Nice wheels!" The young man drove a very sporty bright red Jeep. I was always tickled when Bill noticed and commented on things around him — and demonstrated his undying appreciation for cars and trucks.

The third visit pushed me to my limit. He was applying such force Bill swore at him. There had to be a better way. I felt sick, and sad, as I watched.

Trying to sound calm, I asked, "Paulo, do you realize that by the time you get to your car Bill will have forgotten what you showed him? That by the time you leave our street he will have forgotten you were here?"

To which he gave me *the look* — the now very familiar wife-in-denial look.

As he pulled out of the driveway, I was already on the phone with Bill's case manager.

"I can't stand watching this. I *know* this hurts Bill, and I really don't think this new guy understands the brain aspects of this."

Linda had earned the right to wish to strangle me, but I hoped she understood why I was so critical. Often it was just intuition, but my intuition was based on the sum total of everything that had happened already.

"Can we try someone else?" I asked.

With no discernible impatience, she said, "There isn't anyone else, Catherine. You hated the first two, Cheryl is gone, and the agency just doesn't have anyone else but him in this area."

"Well, then, would it be okay if we just take a short break from it and maybe try again in a few weeks?"

She was agreeable.

Wendy, very skilled in problem solving and improvising, stepped up again, teaching me how to do some passive stretching for the contractures by gradually weighting down Bill's legs.

"This process will require many, many hours, but it will be worth it, if only to keep things from getting worse," she said.

Jan, the PSW, was also proving to be invaluable. I had begun to relax when she was working with Bill, but it struck me as terribly wasteful that she was employed as a personal support worker when so much of her education and experience was in Behavioural Sciences and brain injury. She brought so many new ideas and projects for cognitive work into Bill's life.

One evening she asked, "Could Bill plan his own meals instead of you? We could read the weekly grocery store flyers together and discuss the various foods he would like and make a list for you." It was a brilliant idea that provided a multitude of mind exercises. And saved me from having to do it.

I took the stretching idea Wendy had given me and extended it. During his rest period in the afternoon, I put a pillow on Bill's knees, the over-the-bed table over the pillow, and raised the bed enough to put just a little pressure on his legs. From the end of the bed I pulled gently on his ankles, asking Bill to push his legs straight out. He did this willingly, stretching them a tiny bit at a time.

The idea of putting a rock from the garden on the table occurred to me. I didn't realize at first that it weighed eight kilograms! The instant Bill saw it he called it "Rockin' Ronny." I howled with laughter. A throwback to a teen idol. The rock was forever to be called by that moniker. Bill would grin from ear to ear every time I explained the name to anyone. A lot was happening in his brain.

A LOT WAS happening in my brain, too. Realizing our brief sojourn into the outside world in our own car was over, I slipped a little further into my private cave. Another major success ripped right out from under us. How much more would Bill lose? How much more would we lose?

I still wondered why Cathy Crimmins was so convinced that her American husband, or anyone else, would have quickly or automatically received brain injury rehabilitation in Canada. My husband was born Canadian, served an entire career in the Armed Forces, and paid taxes from his fifteenth birthday, yet it was evident he couldn't get professional rehabilitation. I saw less and less difference between the American and Canadian systems.

24

AN EPIPHANY OF SORTS

On my days off late in May Bill and I tried to get our to-do list finished a little early in the day so we could enjoy our garden. We took many of the exercises and activities outdoors. The electronic pedaller, the Ex N' Flex, worked just as well out on the porch, where we could enjoy the flowers and the fresh warm air. Playing catch and throwing lawn darts was easier and safer outdoors, and throwing toys for Jessie was a wonderful pastime. Bill called her to fetch and chase, honing his fine motor skills as he handed out reward treats.

Still very reluctant to try the Home Care physiotherapist again, but desperate for professional input, I searched the phone book for a therapist who would make house calls. Twenty-one calls. No one made out-of-office visits. Call twenty-two: a private therapist in Belleville who was willing to make house calls. Someone who sounded perfect for Bill. Frank Gielen understood exactly what I was saying about the leg contractures and had an excellent grasp of brain issues. He had previously worked in the system and with people who had brain injuries but had moved to private practice a few years earlier.

When Frank came to meet Bill for the first time, he performed a very thorough assessment, asking many times, "Bill, am I hurting you?" He was gentle, but tested every part of Bill's body and, indirectly, his brain injury status. Bill still took a long time to connect with most new people, but Frank was unconcerned.

His final question to Bill was, "Would you like me to come back to work on some exercises and stretching together, Bill?"

"Sure. Great. See you again."

This was more conversation than Bill had with the previous therapist through three appointments.

A week later, as I put a picture of Frank on the board below "Tuesday, physio day," Bill said, "I remember him."

I was stunned.

"What do you remember about him, Hon?"

"I like him. He's a good guy. Nice dresser. He works hard."

I asked if he preferred Frank to Paulo. Silly question. He didn't remember Paulo.

As weeks went by I watched their relationship grow. Bill liked "the new guy" and didn't object to the work they did, even though it was often difficult and tiring. And work they did. Quickly, I came to see Frank as a much more experienced version of Cheryl. He spoke to Bill as a real participant, even on days when he wasn't participating very much.

Frank, always professional as well as friendly, was never condescending toward me. My endless queries and ideas didn't seem to annoy him, and if they did, he covered it well. Many times he found ways to modify his methods so I could do his exercises with Bill the other days.

Between Frank's visits, the Ex N' Flex pedaller was a daily help, both in strengthening and stretching Bill's arms and legs and in improving his concentration. Once strapped in, he pushed the button to start the machine, which then took his feet and legs through the motion of pedalling with or without effort from him. I set a digital timer. While pedalling, Bill's other task was to check the timer and switch from pedalling forward to backward every two minutes. The more pressure he exerted, the lower the numbers on the monitor went.

We set goals based on the previous sessions and put them on the board to help him to keep track. As his speed increased, so did the value of the exercise. He watched the read-out display and checked the board for his goal number and we both hooted and hollered like children each time he exceeded the previous goal. Thinking, coordination, strength and purpose, all in one workout.

After weeks of this repetitive process, Bill graduated to using hand weights while pedalling, a major accomplishment for someone so poor at multitasking. I loved to see him grin with each new achievement. His enthusiasm waxed and waned at times, but he never refused to do any of the things that would get him "better."

We listened to fiddle music during these workouts. "Helps me get into my rhythm, you know," Bill said. He named each of the Cape Breton fiddlers and recounted stories about the ones he knew. I often fended off tears (happy ones) when I saw him make progress.

KEVIN'S TUESDAYS WITH Bill continued. Apparently the volunteer visitor loved to be tormented and teased. The warmer summer weather allowed them to spend a lot of time out on the deck. On many evenings a ball game erupted, although they only ever used sponge balls, mostly to protect Kevin. Now and then I joined them in three-way catch. It was fascinating to see how fast Bill's reaction time was. The faster Kevin threw the ball to him, the faster he fired it right back. It was often hard to tell which of them enjoyed this more.

There were times, though, when Bill caught the ball, held it, and examined it all over, seeming to contemplate all its details. No amount of coaxing would get him back into the game. Then, without warning, he would fire it at Kevin, smirking. He savoured each time his friend had to go chasing it.

Watching them was another time that I reminded the little devil of those early statements, such as, "This is someone who will never make progress; unlikely to benefit from rehabilitation."

LATE MAY FELT like summer. The unseasonably warm weather gave us more opportunities to expand our life. Many weekends brought company for visits, meals, and pleasant talks. My aunt Loraine, cousin Susan, and her son Adam visited numerous times. Joyce and Earl popped in whenever they could. Brenda was often around to share in social times, too.

Our covered and screened porch meant we could have six or eight for dinner al fresco without enormous effort. Bill was usually in charge of peeling the vegetables. He had definite opinions on what we should serve with what. He had always been the chef in our home and loved to tease me by telling people that cooking was not an area in which I was skilled.

These were pleasant times, even though they were such different times. It was a chance to catch up on family news, world events, and to talk about things other than rehabilitation. Those visits were a blessing for us. Almost like normal.

MUCH OF WENDY'S time in our house included listening to me vent about Home Care problems.

"Why is it so difficult for these agencies to schedule the same person each week? It's only two days a week. Don't they understand how difficult the lack of continuity is for Bill? And for me? Or do they not care?"

My frustration was climbing like the temperature in the desert. Bill's case manager was very competent and understanding, but even she couldn't avert the constant rotation of help. There were so many details, no one person could be expected to grasp them quickly or easily. The biggest obstacle was that it took Bill so long to get comfortable with new people. I seemed to be at odds now with *two* agencies. I could not make them see how detrimental all these new faces were.

I lamented to Linda and Wendy in turn: "I don't understand why we even need nurses for shifts now. Jan, who is a very effective support worker, would be far less costly and is far more useful, in my opinion."

But the system wasn't going to change based on my opinion or our needs.

JUST BEFORE THE beginning of June, I got a call from Terri at the Chedoke Rehab Centre, the same woman who had assessed Bill at the hospital in Trenton almost a year ago.

"How is Bill doing?" she asked. "I hear he's made great progress."

I wondered if Dr. Carlson had been the voice she had heard.

"I am going to be out in your area next week," she continued. "Would it be okay if I dropped by to see you both?"

I was delighted to say yes. I genuinely did want her to come, if only to have her see for herself how much progress Bill had made.

Her visit was, in fact, a mini-assessment. I saw the surprise on her face as she observed all that Bill was doing and how well we were sharing our life at home. That a nursing home had been an outrageous life sentence went unsaid.

"I'm going to do a new report about Bill," she said. "I'm going appeal to the board of directors to get Bill accepted into the 'slow-to-recover' brain injury program. Is that okay with you?"

"Okay?" I asked. "It is so much better than okay."

Assuring me she would do her best but adding she could not promise anything, she shook hands with Bill and departed, taking along a copy of our newest video.

Weeks passed, and gradually my hope faded. But finally Terri did call.

"He's been accepted! Bill can indeed come to Chedoke," she said. Barely pausing for breath, she added, "There will be an opening in October for him."

"Oh, my God! Thank you, Terri. I can't begin to tell you what this will mean for Bill, for both of us. I can only imagine how much he will gain from this!"

Finally, the heath care system was going to work for Bill.

The Chedoke Centre was the very place where Walter Gretzky had gone for rehabilitation. Through his book I had learned a lot about it and its one-on-one therapists. In spite of the ongoing problems and frustrations I soared with optimism about our life and Bill's new future. We started every morning with a kiss and hug, and every night we went to sleep in the warmth and comfort of each other's arms. I wanted October to arrive tomorrow.

IN AUGUST AND September we were able to use the local wheelchair transport services several times to venture downtown to the local Show 'n Shine car show. Bill had owned a classic car for years and was still very keen on them. As I wheeled him around, he would exclaim, "Look at that paint job! I had a '64 just like that. See that red one? The guy's a jerk and his car is junk."

Frequently, we encountered fellows who had known Bill for years. They usually moved away from us as fast as they dared. I bristled at their discomfort, asking myself why men were such pansies about disabilities. These outings, while not my favourite activity, were wonderful for both of us: Bill loved the cars, the trucks, the outdoors. I just loved that we were out together.

Between the marvels of progress were still lots of days that were less than stellar. These were getting farther and farther apart, though. Some days Bill was way below par, some days just a little below, some days he was amazing. There was rarely a clear reason for these variations. Sometimes it was energy level. Other times an infection was lurking. Sometimes there had been too much stimulation. Other times not enough.

I had slowly accepted that we would never regain our former life. An epiphany of sorts for me. I was coming to see this chapter of our life as the true benchmark of our love and values. Would I have preferred him to have bypassed all these issues? Absolutely. Did I ever consider that the nursing home would have been a better solution? Absolutely not.

25

DEFINITELY NOT HOMEY

Finally, a week before Thanksgiving, the day arrived to go to the Chedoke Rehabilitation Centre. I loaded our cargo, including the most important items: his photo album, *Bill's Home Care Book*, including his daily schedule and medications and the pages on his daily activities. There was a lot to know about him.

We left at nine in the morning, knowing it would be at least a three-hour trip, provided there were no traffic jams along the way. Getting into the car was much harder since he had developed the leg contractures, but it was worth every ounce of effort to be able to travel in our own car.

Bill kept up a running commentary about the cows, farms, and cars and trucks we passed. One truck in particular caught his attention.

"That Kenworth is from Quebec. What do you think he has on board?" he asked, pointing to a livestock carrier.

"Cows, maybe?"

"Poor cows, then. They're on their last road trip."

Several times he put his head back and closed his eyes either to drift off or block out my driving.

My thoughts drifted off, too. I was remembering what I had read in Walter Gretzky's book about his rehabilitation and stroke recovery at Chedoke. He was transferred there once his medical condition stabilized. He was candid about his situation, including specific information about his speech and memory problems. He wrote about how long it had taken before he could walk on his own, and how he had progressed to that point only after many, many hours of therapists supporting him physically on every step.

Walter credited his recovery, in large part, to the young man who worked as his one-on-one therapist. They plotted out his day in minute detail and made a chart of the many things he had to relearn. He also needed to relearn most of his own history.

I had borrowed that day plan and put it to work for Bill. Walter's therapist had worked with him for hours each day, every day of the week, struggling right along with him to find ways to help him progress. Physio and cognitive therapies were part of his daily routine. Each element of his day was done in a repetitive, consistent way. I had borrowed that chart of his schedule, adjusting it to suit our situation and time frame. Some days Walter was willing and able. Some days he was uncooperative and difficult.

The book talked about how important his family had been in his recovery and improvement, how he couldn't have done it alone. It was a beautiful story, honest and direct. Walter's book reiterated that time was a big factor: That the earlier the intervention, the greater the scope for improvement. It seemed like so long ago now that his story and experience had given me the template to start our own program, however basic and amateur.

I chuckled to myself at my naïveté back then. It had never crossed my mind then, or even in the months to follow, that it would take twenty months to finally get quality rehabilitation for Bill. Not here in Canada, here where our system is so much better than the American system. Not here, where the "experts" know how important early intervention is.

Bill brought me back from my meanderings.

"How about ice cream?"

"What kind?" I inquired, smiling. I already knew the answer.

He thought, and thought, and thought.

"Vanilla! I know — I'm boring about ice cream."

I squeezed his hand and laughed. A running joke of ours for years had been about his going to ice cream shops that sold fifty-two flavours and almost always ordering vanilla.

We got our ice cream at a drive-through, and between licks and drips, our conversation turned back to our destination.

"This is going to be a wonderful experience for you, Hon. The staff at the centre are experts in the stuff you are doing. Maybe not the boxing, but I'm sure they will have activities that are more advanced than what we can do at home. You will have some fun with the other people too, I bet, once you get to know them. What do you think?"

He looked over at me, and I saw a shadow of uncertainty in his eyes. My heart lurched. Was he feeling the same anxiety I was? I could barely stand to think about him being there without me. For at least the tenth time I said, "Well, this is the place Wayne Gretzky's dad came to for help."

He was intrigued, as if this was the first he had heard of this.

"Is he still there?"

"No, he got much better and went home and continued working at home, just like you will."

"Are you really sure about that?"

"I am positive."

"Okay, I love you."

"Love you, too."

Bill drifted off to sleep again, and I went back to daydreaming about highly skilled staff working with Bill on leg strengthening and straightening, weight bearing, and a multitude of brain injury problems. I prayed they would have and use a standing frame. One of my biggest regrets was not being able to buy one for him, knowing what a difference it would have made. I was excited he would finally get real help. He was willing to work hard and wanted to keep improving.

This helped ease my qualms, a little, about leaving him alone in the care of strangers. I chided myself. "Stop it, Cath. This is what you screamed and begged for this past year and a half! These people are professionals. They know their business. They will take care of him."

Finally in the parking lot, we disembarked without incident. The question of baggage was easily solved. Once Bill was in his chair, I piled everything on him as if he were a packhorse. I had been showing him the picture of him with Terri for two weeks. She was familiar to him now, and when she greeted him warmly, he smiled and said hello as if she were more than a casual acquaintance. In fact, Bill enjoyed seeing Terri. He loved attention from tall, beautiful young women, and she was all that, and warm and caring as well.

Terri ushered us to his room in the slow-to-recover section. This program had only five participants, three in Bill's room and two others in the room next door. She introduced us to a couple of the nurses, then gave us some time to get Bill settled.

Only then did I start to take in the details of his new space. I thought there must have been a huge sale years ago on dull grey-green paint, because the colour of the walls was the same as that of the Complex Continuing Care unit in the Trenton Hospital. His new room looked gloomy and drab, depressing really, with fluorescent lighting and grey-green curtains on the windows.

Bill would be sharing his space with two other men. There were three beds, each with its own chair and metal table, each in a corner. The fourth corner housed a metal table, four narrow closets, a sink, a large garbage pail, two chairs, and some medical equipment. A TV sat atop a portable stand, blaring. I reached over and turned it off.

Each bed had a curtain that could be pulled right around. This would help, I thought, since Bill was still having three in/out catheters every day. At least he would have some privacy. It was not cheerful, not uplifting, definitely not homey. But, I reminded myself, "We're not here for the décor; we're here for the expertise and help."

As I hung up his clothes, put away his toiletries, and used the shelves for the hand weights, cylinders, and balls we had brought, I reminded Bill this was not going to be a very long stay.

"Only a few weeks to a couple of months probably, Hon. Just think about all the different stuff you will get to work on and all the progress you'll make. Be back to your old self in no time."

"I sure hope so." His voice was subdued.

"This will be great, and you get a break from me harassing you!" I struggled to keep my voice confident, encouraging, and enthusiastic. I was feeling subdued, too.

"I sure hope so," he repeated, but his expression was as flat as his voice.

Suddenly, a wheelchair raced over to us from across the room. A man, one of his roommates, I assumed, was extremely interested in the new guy. In fact, he never took his eyes off Bill. He got as close as his wheels allowed and peered into Bill's face, seeming to take in every detail. He said nothing, but continued to lean in and stare.

We were both a little taken aback. Bill did not like strangers getting this close. I was fairly sure there was no harm in this situation, but Bill looked less certain. Suddenly, without warning, the man turned his wheelchair and raced (as much as you can in a chair) out the door and down the hallway.

Just a few moments later we both became acutely aware of strange noises across the room. The curtains had just been opened, and there lay the other roommate.

A nurse reported to me later, "This poor fellow suffered a massive stroke many months ago. He can't speak or move any of his limbs himself. He has severe contractures in all four limbs."

The nurse also mentioned that his wife was here most of the

time. I hoped this nurse didn't share that much private information about every patient with strangers.

Good God, in comparison with this man, we had fared so much better. The man was being tube-fed and could move only his eyes. He couldn't speak at all, but the sounds he emitted gave a voice to his desperate state. He was frequently attended to by nurses coming and going. I heard my mother's voice reminding me, "There is always someone with a greater problem."

Doubt was already rearing its head. How would this environment affect Bill? This was not the cheery, comfortable atmosphere he had at home. Was this place going to encourage and motivate him? Or would he fear he was going to end up the same? When I left to go back to the city, would he think I had abandoned him? That he was staying here forever?

A nurse came in to take Bill's vitals. She didn't seem particularly friendly and didn't seem to notice that Bill was a person, not just a body, but she was efficient. I was puzzled that she spoke only to me. Never directly to Bill. Again I quickly reminded myself, "Oh well, Cath, he's not here for nursing. Stop worrying!"

Just past noon we met the physiotherapist, an easy-going woman named Beverley. I relaxed a little as she asked questions about Bill and included him in the conversation. Beverley then explained what the program involved and said she would work with Bill every other day for an hour or so and assess his progress.

Every other day for an hour? I felt queasy again. My main goal all along had been to get extensive physio for Bill. I had always believed and hoped that, as he gained back his strength and became more able physically, he would also make giant leaps cognitively. He had already proved himself at home. Two or three hours a week? This was not what I had expected.

I asked a few questions, filled her in on his activities, and mentioned that Bill communicated very well at home but was much more reticent with strangers. I squeezed his hand, more to get support *from* him than to give it.

Beverley stood up to leave, shook hands with each of us, and promised to see us in the morning to get started.

Bill and I decided to go outside, tour the grounds, and get some fresh air. We needed an escape.

When we returned to his room, a nurse came to explain the lunch and supper routine. Patients must go to the dining room unless they were sick. Not negotiable. Well, that made sense to me. I wanted Bill to continue to see himself as healthy and here to get therapy, not medical attention.

Travelling down the hallway, we stopped to enjoy some of the lovely paintings on the wall. Someone had tried hard to make this public area less depressing. Good for them.

As I inspected a landscape, Bill peeked into the room beside his and saw two very young men in stretcher chairs staring blankly at the world. Seemingly, neither of them could move anything, even their eyes. They looked to be comatose.

Bill exhaled loudly, saying, "Oh my God."

That said it all for me, too.

"Aren't we lucky, Hon? All you need to do is get your legs straight and strong. These people have a very long, tough road ahead of them."

"For sure," he agreed, sounding skeptical about their possible progress.

As we entered the dining room, I gasped. I knew this centre was for both amputees and brain injury patients, but this scene looked like a hospital in a World War II movie for horribly maimed and psychologically impaired soldiers.

There were at least six rows of tables placed end to end running horizontal to the small self-serve food area at the front of the large, grey windowless room. Those who could had to pick up their own meal. Logical. Most would need to be able to do this in the outside world. Someone brought trays to those who couldn't. There were all manner of amputations in sight: missing arms, missing legs — several people were missing two limbs.

Guilt over my reaction rolled over me. I was grateful that this facility and its staff were here to help people learning to cope with such life-changing situations, but, oh my God...

A pleasant kitchen worker showed us to what would be Bill's seat while he was here. The other five assigned to his table were already in place. Not one was able to feed himself. Each one had a caregiver for the task, and they were doing it for them, not assisting them. I struggled to control my expression. Mostly so Bill wouldn't pick up on my reaction.

Once positioned at the table, Bill's gaze travelled to each person across from him, then down the rows of tables, lingering on each face. He dropped his eyes and stared blankly at the placemat in front of him. It had his name and room number on it and a note about his fruit allergy.

"Are you okay, Hon?" I asked.

No answer.

Watching an attendant feeding the person across from us, spilling as much as she spooned, I asked Bill, "Would you like to move?"

An emphatic nod.

"Okay, let's go."

I rushed him out of his designated space. We were stopped at the end of the table by the nice lady who had seated us. She asked where we were going.

"We're going to another table."

"You really can't do that."

"Well, actually, we can. Just watch."

I headed to an empty table at the back of the room and positioned Bill with his back to the others. Staring at a blank wall would be better than seeing the rest of this room. In a quiet voice, hoping to lift Bill's spirits, I again remarked on how fortunate we were to have such small problems compared with this group. I was met with another skeptical look.

Bill picked at the food on his plate; obviously his appetite had been soured. We left before dessert. Down a hallway we found a lounge, complete with TV and pool table. We agreed to come back there tomorrow to see if Bill could reach the tabletop and try a game of 9-ball.

I helped Bill get ready for and into bed. Grudgingly, after some persuading, the evening nurse had brought his pills and done his catheter to accommodate his normal schedule. I wondered if scheduling would be an issue here, too. It had always seemed ludicrous, even cruel, to wake someone up in the middle of the night for this very invasive task. It seemed to me every institution scheduled things for staff convenience rather than patient well-being.

With the curtain still drawn, I climbed onto the bed and curled up in Bill's arms. We hugged, and hugged, and hugged. In a whisper I said, "You'll only be here for a short time, Hon, and mostly I'll be here, too. We can do this, can't we?"

A whisper came back: "I don't know."

IT WAS DARK outside, and I needed to find my lodgings. I tried to sound reassuring and confident as I put on my jacket.

"I'll be back here before you wake up, and I know you will be just fine. I love you so much."

"I wubs you, too."

That old joke of ours. He tried to muster a smile.

I was barely outside the door when the tears started flowing down my face. Was he feeling as sad and fearful as I was?

26
ATTACK AND RETREAT

A VERY UNCOMFORTABLE BED in a very crummy hotel near the centre guaranteed my early arrival the next morning. Before dawn I was sitting beside Bill's bed again, there when he woke up, as promised.

I sneaked breakfast into his room and added his cereal from home to the tray. The day nurse was mildly critical about this breach of the meal rules.

"The hell with you. This is my husband, and I know the impact that dining room will have on him. Nothing good." I did not let this thought out of my mouth. I just nodded and grunted, "Mmhmm."

Mid-morning the young staff doctor introduced himself. First name Rob, surname unpronounceable. I introduced him to Bill as Dr. Rob. Did the doctor bristle? His body language told me he expected to be addressed formally. Too bad.

He checked Bill over and listened to his chest. He frowned and listened again. I started to explain that Bill had suffered severe pneumonia many years ago, that he had almost died, and that now, every time anyone listened to his chest, they heard a phantom problem. I suggested he might find that in the records from our family doctor.

After continuing to ignore me a few more minutes, he took his leave. When he was out of the room, Bill said, "Asshole." I agreed totally.

Late morning the recreational therapist arrived, a nice friendly gal. We discussed some of Bill's goals, and she explained some of the routines. I was shocked when she said, "Friday afternoons the staff take the slow-to-recover patients on a field trip."

"A field trip?"

"Yes, we take them on an excursion in a wheelchair-accessible bus. We go to see the local castle, the Botanical Gardens, movies, or sometimes to the mall."

"Are you kidding me? At best you have two of five people in this program who might even begin to take in new surroundings, and you haul them somewhere to entertain them? This must take at least five staff, plus the expense of transportation and whatever else."

God knows I was trying not to sound harsh.

"Bill is living proof that being in as normal an environment as possible has incredible value, but going out to a movie with total strangers, in a strange city, without me, does not feel right. I'm sorry, but under no circumstances is Bill to be included in these outings."

Thoughts were galloping through my mind by now. "Who is running the asylum? Who thinks up these things? Here, in a rehabilitation centre, I was expecting people to work with him on the things we don't already know and do."

Later in the morning, the occupational therapist came in. We talked about the dining room issues, and, although she didn't necessarily agree with me, she understood my fears. We struck a deal: For two weeks, because I would be there most days, Bill could have his meals in his room or the lounge, but after that he must go to the dining room. She did offer to come in and have lunch with Bill herself when I was at work. That was reassuring.

We went over the pertinent problems we were struggling with. Initiation was the biggest one. Bill was most obliging when anyone asked him to do anything, but often he couldn't get started without a cue. It would give him much more freedom from being directed and nagged if he could master that lost ability. Conversations, especially on the phone, were very tough for him because of this.

I went over some of my frustration about getting Home Care people to help Bill only as needed, and said I hoped that here he would become more able to do things in sequence on his own, even if it required a chart or list. This would of course spill over into most aspects of his daily life. She nodded, appearing to understand our goals.

After lunch, we started doing our normal afternoon activities, but I soon realized we were disrupting the man and his wife in the other corner. It was a bright, cool fall day, just a few days until Thanksgiving, so outside we went. Bill carried the sponge balls, cylinders, and our photo album. I pushed. The grounds were quite pretty once you got to the back of the building, almost park like. We tossed the balls, wandered to different areas, sneaked some kisses, and clung to each other, physically and emotionally.

Beverley, the physiotherapist, was waiting for us when we got back. She took Bill to the gym and got to work. First they did a pivot transfer from Bill's chair to a platform. He was not very helpful. I could see how unsure he was of this stranger. Beverley helped him lie down and checked his leg contractures. We showed her the routine he had for rolling, shifting position, and sitting up again.

I could see that this woman knew her work. Part of her approach was similar to Frank's, which buoyed my confidence. Next they headed for the Ex N' Flex pedaller. I asked Bill to show Beverley how he went through his exercise regimen. He looked at me and didn't move a muscle. A casual observer would have bet he'd never even seen this machine before. It took three minutes to get him started, and longer to get him doing what he always did.

Beverley was able to get an idea of the patterns we followed for direction change and increase and decrease of pressure and the rest. I wondered if Bill would, in fact, do this for her.

Back in Bill's room, the nonverbal man was watching the television, which was blaring; the other patient was moaning non-stop. I pulled the curtain around us while Bill had supper. But long before I was ready, I knew it was time for me to leave. With much holding and hugging, I reminded him I'd only be a few blocks away and would be there when he woke up. Bill looked dejected and forlorn, which was exactly how I felt.

LEAVING THE PARKING lot I ran the day's events through my mind. I berated myself for not having asked many more questions about the program here. I wondered about the difference between "regular" and "slow-to-recover" brain injury rehabilitation. With only a few hour-long sessions of physiotherapy a week, Bill was sure to be slow to recover.

I thought about the other four people currently in this program: Bob, the stroke victim, lay in a bed twenty-four hours a day. He was having Botox injections in his limbs and therapy to stretch those limbs every day. Otherwise, not much else was being done at this point. The two young men in the next room seemed to be on about the same regimen, with neither of them being able to speak or move their limbs. I hadn't seen any therapists working with the fourth man, although I presumed they did. Completely nonverbal, but slightly more advanced physically than Bill, he could at least get into his wheelchair alone to race around.

Already I was wishing that Bill were in a *not-so-slow-to-recover* program. Of course that had never been offered, ever, by anyone.

It was very dark, raining lightly, and a gusty wind was blowing wet leaves all over the roads. A staff member had suggested I try getting a room at a nearby convent, which had been converted to a retreat and conference centre. It was closer and less expensive. Driving around a strange city in the dark looking for the place was infuriating, and I was overreacting. I cursed out every driver in front of and behind me, yelled (though only inside the car) at the pedestrian who stepped off the curb without looking, and generally worked myself into a fury.

Finally I found the retreat house. Even in the darkness the grounds were truly beautiful. The front yard was a glorious old-world garden. It looked like an antebellum plantation. I wandered to a wet garden seat, sank down onto it, and sobbed and sobbed and sobbed.

"How could one woman be so emotional?" I thought. "You need to smarten up, be positive, lose the neurotic thoughts, and be grateful. You have to do this, for Bill's sake, no matter what it takes. You cannot blow his only chance for rehab."

27

GOING AWOL

WEDNESDAY DAWNED BRIGHT AND a little warmer. Bill was awake when I arrived, and a nurse was getting his clothes out of the closet. She brought over a shirt and a pair of pants that didn't go well together.

"Did Bill choose those?" I asked, quite sure he would never have combined those colours.

"No, I just grabbed the first things in there. I need to get him ready quickly. It's going to be a busy day."

Trying to sound cheerful, I asked, "Why don't I do that with him, since I'm here and not really doing anything else?"

She was happy to have less to do, and I was happy to start over, following our home routine to get his day underway. We started with his choosing what he wanted to wear. He chose navy and powder blue.

Our day was interrupted only once. The occupational therapist came to have lunch with Bill. She just observed, without drawing attention to anything, and only after Bill had finished did she offer any comments. She had some ideas she would try over the next days and offered to keep me apprised. I valued her suggestions and especially appreciated that she would share lunchtime with Bill. But I still had concerns about the other meals. How would the nurses approach this?

Far too soon, it was time for me to leave. Really leave. I had a three-hour drive back to Trenton ahead of me, and another long one to work in the city the next morning. It was a very difficult goodbye. I wrote a reminder on Bill's whiteboard: "Cath will be back on Friday afternoon."

"It's really only a day and a half. I will leave work really early and come straight here to get you. It's Thanksgiving this weekend and we need to get home to celebrate."

I laughed, smiled, and acted light-hearted, hugging and kissing my husband. Drawing myself out of his arms, I backed out of the room. I made it to the car before the tears flowed.

I CALLED MORNING and night on Thursday, and again early Friday morning. The nursing staff were not as willing to give me information as the staff at Kingston General had been. I got only the bare essentials. He was fine. No, they didn't know which therapists he had seen. No, they didn't know what else he had done.

I would have to devise a better means of communicating for the future.

My sense of loss being away from Bill was intense, and I truly hoped it was less so for him. I considered trying to rent a cheap room near the centre for the coming months where I could bring Jessie. Bill's stay would likely be fewer than five or six months. We'd be together so much more.

The extra traffic at the beginning of a long weekend turned the normal hour-and-a-half drive from Toronto into a four-hour nerve-wracking trek, and my arrival in Bill's room didn't provide me with the reception I expected. Bill didn't want to kiss me. Or to hug me. That was a first.

I'd been promised by the neurologist who was overseeing this program that there would be no medication changes without discussing them with me. As we gathered our things for the weekend, though, a nurse came by with Bill's weekend pills. There was an extra package. One I didn't recognize.

"I don't think these are for Bill," I said.

"Yes, they are."

She named the medication. I had never heard of it. Rather than argue with the nurse I decided our pharmacist would be my first call in the morning.

With his weekend luggage on his lap I pushed Bill to the car. Just as I was half in and half out of the back seat stashing his belongings, Bill took the brakes off his chair. I hadn't realized we were on a slight slope. He was taking a joy ride. As I ran to catch him, I cursed myself for not asking for help from the staff. I thanked the parking lot gods for no moving vehicles.

The five-hour drive back to Trenton, on a long weekend, made the venture tiring. But worse, Bill was withdrawn. Not speaking. Was he mad at me? Had something happened?

SAFELY BACK HOME, though, it was worth all the effort for the reception Bill got. Jessie went crazy. The hairy little white fur ball launched herself onto his lap. She licked him, burrowed into his jacket, and leaped up and down on him. He in turn laughed his heart out, enjoying her affection and attention. This was worth crawling over shards of glass for. Jessie seemed to be the only thing that cheered him up on Saturday. I missed our normal chatter.

On Sunday morning the pharmacist explained the pills Bill had been given were for intestinal issues, which Bill didn't have. They were not for urinary tract issues, which he did have. The pharmacist also cautioned that, although they were herbal products, they were not suitable for anyone taking blood thinners, which Bill did. Bloody wonderful.

Company came to visit that day, and we did what we could of our normal routines over the weekend, but both of us were in slow mode and Bill seemed to have lost his focus. All the travelling had taken a toll, so we just relaxed during the evenings. We watched some TV and cuddled in bed, all three of us. Sleeping curled up together was always such a soothing experience.

MONDAY AFTERNOON WE embarked on our return to Chedoke. The rainy weather and extra holiday traffic made it another five-hour journey, but we had time to talk about the coming week. Bill was quiet for long periods and seemed to be retreating again. I continued to reassure him the week would bring lots of new, good experiences.

"Are you sure?"

"Positive."

When I put the car in park Bill finally spoke again.

"Let's just go home, please?"

I wanted desperately to do just that, but I persuaded him we needed to give this more time.

Back in his room, I noticed the garbage pail was full to overflowing. Syringes and used gloves lay on the table. The floor was dirty. I unpacked his personal belongings and stored them on the shelves, trying to make light of the surroundings. Once Bill was back in his bed he seemed to deflate even more.

And then the clock struck nine, and I had to leave him again. I wrote on his board: "I'm just down the road. I will be here when you wake up. I love you."

Again I found myself drawn to the peaceful gardens at the retreat house. The Sister on night duty came out to see me. Accustomed to providing lodging to people connected with Chedoke, she chatted quietly with me, wanting to know more about our story. Once I started, I spilled out the lot: Bill's fears, my fears, and my loss of faith in our system.

"Just sit here quietly, dear, and pray," she said. "God will guide you."

"I am always trying to make deals with God."

"No, dear, ask Him for guidance, not a deal, and He will give it."

EARLY THE NEXT morning I stood outside the curtain around the bed, and eavesdropped. The nurse had brought his clothes and was saying, "Bill, I'm going to get you washed and shaved and dressed, and then get you up into your wheelchair with the lift."

I stepped inside the curtain and quietly said, "You know, at home Bill does most of his own showering and shaving, and he chooses his own clothes for the day. Then he gets himself dressed. He requires some assistance, but mostly just guidance. Then he does a pivot transfer with me to the chair."

"I didn't even know he could sit up on his own," she said.

Bill was listening, but wouldn't look up at me, or her. He looked disheartened.

After breakfast, as we waited for the physiotherapist, the occupational therapist arrived.

"No, today isn't his day for physiotherapy," she said. "This week physiotherapy will be only twice because of the holiday."

That was the proverbial straw that broke my silence.

"The equivalent of less than three hours of physiotherapy and a few hours of occupational therapy per week isn't going to help Bill. In fact, what he didn't do at home these past ten days already shows. I am sorry, and I know I must seem really difficult, but this is just not what I expected."

I was speaking quietly, but with authority. I wasn't exactly angry, but I certainly was frustrated. And afraid.

The therapist departed quickly.

A short time later a social worker appeared — summoned by the therapist, I assumed. As we talked, I tried to conceal my general distrust of folks in her occupation. In my experience they hadn't proved very helpful. Sitting by a window just outside Bill's room, sniffling and sobbing, I could barely form full sentences.

"We didn't go through all this to get here, to Chedoke, so Bill could do Ex N' Flex twice a week. He does so much more than this at home with our amateur stuff. I thought he'd get so much more and much more superior therapy here."

Blowing my nose between sniffles, I blurted out, "I thought there would be a lot more therapy, more like Walter Gretzky wrote about. This seems so damned wasteful, and Bill is regressing every day. Not progressing. My expectations were unrealistic, I guess. Again."

Where was all the rehabilitation Walter Gretzky talked about in his book? How did I get it so wrong, again?

Miss Social Worker placated, sympathized, and commiserated, but she had no practical suggestions.

I was free falling into despair again. I needed to talk to someone who would really understand. I took a chance and, when Bill was resting, called Dr. Peter Carlson, the neuropsychologist at the Regional Community Brain Injury Services office in Kingston. He was familiar with our challenges, the progress Bill had already made at home, and my intuitions about Bill. He had been part of the process of getting Bill accepted into this special program.

He listened to my recitation of the already obvious negative changes in Bill, and my fears about how much more ground he could, and likely would, lose by being here.

Sobbing, I asked him, "Does 'slow to recover' really mean 'considered hopeless'? Because that's how three of the four other patients in this program seem."

He had a few of his own questions and patiently waited for me to stop sniffling and answer them. I thought I could hear him taking a deep breath before he spoke.

"Catherine, you know Bill better than anyone. You have always put what you believe is best for him above anyone else's opinion. Don't stop now. If you believe this is compromising him, and he isn't going to get what he needs without a lot of regression, follow your instincts. They have served you both very well so far. If going home feels like the right thing to do, then do it. Go home."

The Sister at the retreat house was right. I had asked God to guide me to what was truly right for Bill, and now a professional whose opinion I valued and respected was reaffirming my ability to judge these circumstances and their negative impact on Bill.

First stop was the nursing station to announce we were leaving that very day. I apologized to as many people as I could, but stood firm. We couldn't afford the two or more weeks it would take for them to get to know Bill and his abilities. Every day was a setback. Everyone suggested I give it a longer try, but I was too afraid he would regress even more.

"No, thank you. We really must be going," I said as if I were declining tea.

Packing up took no time at all. I stuffed Bill's things into bags like a whirling dervish. He was bewildered, but when I asked if he would prefer to go home and get back to work with Frank, he said, "Affirmative!"

28

TEAMWORK

IT WAS A RELIEF to be back home, together. The Chedoke exercise in futility had taken a toll on both of us. Bill's regression was significant. Getting back on track and regaining all that lost progress seemed impossible to me. I was discouraged and afraid, having lost all hope that Bill would ever get the help he really needed. I wondered now if that help even existed, except perhaps in Walter Gretzky's world.

Although Dr. Carlson had reassured me that my decision to take Bill out of Chedoke wouldn't stand in the way of future opportunities at another rehab program, that wasn't much comfort. What other opportunities were there? If other programs were possible, why hadn't they been offered already?

It took a few days for the whole experience to sink in and a few more for our emotions to dissipate. We talked about all the ups and downs of being away from home and agreed we weren't cut out for it.

"Do you think I'm becoming a control freak?"

He laughed at that.

"What do you mean, 'becoming'?" Then he said, "I wubs you."

I felt tears welling up. This silly phrase he had always used when I was feeling unsure of myself and needed propping up still worked wonders. That so little of his pre-brain-problem personality had changed was a reminder of why we were doing all this together.

"I wubs you, too!" I offered gratefully.

WENDY CONTINUED TO support both of us, but at times, now, it seemed to be more about me than Bill. I was teetering on the edge of the abyss again, angry much of the time.

"Why couldn't he have been given the opportunity for *proper* rehabilitation early on?" I asked her. "How much does he have to do to prove he has potential? What the hell is 'slow to recover' anyway? Is that just a term for 'oops, we let him fall through the cracks'? How many more people does he have to adjust to? How much more training of people will it take to get the message across that he isn't going to die this week?"

Wendy continued to encourage me.

"You need to take a breath, look around, and accept that this place, your home, is where you are both most comfortable and secure. Bill is where he is now because of what you two do together. What you are to each other. Better days will be back."

BY THE FIRST week of November 2004, most of the leaves had fallen. Our garden was awash in multicoloured leaves. On a crisp, bright, orangey kind of Sunday I looked outside and asked Bill, "Do you want to just get out and enjoy an autumn day?"

He was all for it so we put our routine aside and headed outside. Bill laughed as Jessie dived into the piles of leaves I raked, scattering them back almost to their original location. Seeing him enjoy her and watching her hairy little body diving in and out of the rustling brown, yellow, and orange leaves gave me a great lift. As I raked,

Bill held the bag so I could deposit my gatherings in it. We made eye contact. We understood each other implicitly: *This is what we love to do together. Life is good. Not the same as before, but very good. Perspective is everything.*

JAN WAS BACK on the schedule immediately, which was amazing, as we had expected to be gone for many weeks, if not months. Theresa, our favourite visiting nurse, continued her weekly visits to assess Bill. She was always so careful and conscientious with him. She monitored medical details, but there wasn't much to worry about right now. Theresa understood why I got so frustrated and fatigued by the constant change of home care nurses, and she recommended I request a new, young graduate nurse, Susan, a girl she thought would be very well suited to Bill and our home program.

It took weeks to get to meet her, but Susan was everything Theresa had said. Perhaps it was her newness to the profession that made her so open and willing to learn about Bill as an individual. She wasn't deterred by my litany of information, either. She was excited and enthusiastic. No sign of being jaded or presumptuous.

She connected with Bill on her very first visit. I took pictures of them together and one of Susan alone for Bill's photo album, hoping they would be much used in the future. I was anxious to get her slotted in for my workdays. Intuitively, and because of Bill's response to her, I had a very positive feeling about her, but, as was so often the case, it would still take months to get her scheduled consistently with Bill.

The first morning that she was coming to work with Bill, I printed her name on his whiteboard. As I put her picture up, Bill put on a smile as wide as a canyon, showing as many teeth as he could. His eyes were twinkling when he said, "Miss Teeth." Susan was a small girl with an enormous smile. She had very big teeth, white and shiny. It was encouraging that he remembered her so clearly after just one meeting.

Soon after we went AWOL from Chedoke, Wendy came up with

a new opportunity. She spelled it out for Bill and me.

"There is a college program called Behavioural Sciences. Students learn how to work with people with a variety of life issues, including addictions, mental illness, and brain injury. The students need practice time as part of their credits."

She told Bill about a young woman who wanted to do her practical segment with him through Regional Community Brain Injury Services.

"Understanding how to develop a unique plan for an individual is paramount in this course, and Michele would be perfect for you. Would you like to take part, Bill?"

"Oh sure, what the hell," Bill answered.

Wendy glanced at me to see if I was in accord, knowing how pleased I would be that Bill had made his own decision.

"If Bill is in, I'm in."

Michele joined Bill's team in November. She was bright, funny, and interested in Bill. I took a photo of her with Wendy and Bill the first day we met her, hoping it would help Bill connect the dots: Bill plus Wendy = Michele.

Before Michele arrived for her first workday with Bill, I put the picture on the whiteboard.

"Last week they came to visit us," I said. "Michele is coming to work with you. She has some great ideas to make your workouts more fun."

When he saw the photo he seemed to remember her.

To get Michele started, I demonstrated the approach we took every morning to orient Bill to his day. First thing was to determine the day and date and write it on his whiteboard. It always went something like, "If yesterday was Sunday, November 3, what day is today?"

Most days I got the correct answer, but some days not. I took it as a good sign when he gave the right answer that morning. He finally seemed to be recalling the details. Another reminder of the need for repetition. He demonstrated lots of the things he did best. The very first day he outdid himself. He was actually showing off.

For the first few days Michele spent her time just getting to know Bill as a person as well as his strengths and weaknesses.

Michele's work involved developing strategies with Wendy. One of the biggest obstacles was Bill's inability to attend. His mind wandered. He would at times lose focus, get bored, or simply forget what he was doing. I was eager to have someone knowledgeable try a new approach. As the days rolled by I felt the need to intervene less and less. Bill had made a real connection with Michele and they were accomplishing new things. Several weeks into her assignment I videotaped their progress.

The new video was a major success. Michele was coaching Bill to volley his giant fit ball back and forth across the room to her. "Bill, can you hit it back with your left hand?" He did. "How about with your right hand?" He did. "Okay, great. Now can you volley it back with both hands?"

As the volleys continued, Michele kicked the pace up a notch and asked for hand changes randomly. She asked for a right-hand volley three times in a row, threw in one left-hand throw, and then one or two with both hands. Now and again she had to repeat a specific change several times before he would make the switch.

They moved on to kicking a big ball back and forth to one another. He put his feet up on top of the ball, balancing himself on the bed. (This is not an easy exercise for an able-bodied, or able-minded, person. For a patient with a brain injury it was very challenging.) Pushing with all his might, Bill sent the ball across the room to Michele.

I marvelled again that we had been told this man was never going to be able even to sit up on his own, much less be able to enjoy a life in our home with me.

Now, reaching forward and down to pick up various cylinders as Michele requested them, Bill responded to her instructions flawlessly. We did this together all the time, but now he was doing it with someone else. As I watched, from my out-of-the-way corner, a wave of sadness washed over me. I rarely saw Bill through any but the most optimistic of eyes. But here, behind a camera, I began to see what a stranger would see.

Yes, he was very much compromised. But would strangers, even those who had come to know us through the agencies, understand this was *so much more* than he would ever have had in a nursing home? Would they wonder, as I did, how much more might have been attained had he been given the chance to get real therapy in real rehab programs with properly trained specialists? Would they understand this was the best place for us, in spite of the problems that inevitably popped up?

JAN, THE PSW, continued to develop a special relationship with Bill. They bantered back and forth, and he truly enjoyed his time with her. One night she told me a story.

"Bill was unusually slow eating his dinner at the table tonight, and I was just keeping him company. He noticed I wasn't eating and took a piece of chicken from his own plate and placed it gently onto mine. I guess he forgot I had already eaten my meal. He was so thoughtful. When I said, 'No, Bill, it's yours, you eat it,' he answered, 'No, please, I really want to share it with you.'"

A lump formed in my throat and tears pooled in Jan's eyes. My Bill was still in there, through and through.

While Jan, Michele, Theresa, and, whenever possible, Susan were doing their utmost for us, and doing it very well, agency conflicts were still part of life. Poor communication and my intolerance were rearing up again. Susan told me a number of times she was very interested in working the daytime shifts every Thursday and Friday, but for some reason, she wasn't being scheduled for them routinely.

Wendy offered to put together a mini-meeting. She thought perhaps if everyone involved in Bill's case had a better understanding of acquired brain injury, it might help them to grasp my constant concerns about the perpetual cycle of new home care staff. I was very encouraged by her idea. Coming from me, the information didn't seem to reach the right people. I often felt, correctly or otherwise, that the agency people saw me as a difficult, demanding, and unreasonable wife. Sometimes they were right.

29

TUESDAYS WITH BILL

In attendance at the help-in-our-home meeting were Wendy and Michele, the student from RCBIS; Linda, our Home Care case manager from CCAC; Jan and the other personal support worker, as well as their agency supervisor; Theresa, Susan, and one other shift nurse; as well as the nursing agency's manager. It was a full house.

Wendy gave a very concise overview of the brain, complete with pictures, showing exactly where Bill's brain had sustained trauma from the surgery and tumour. She described how damage to the arousal centre caused Bill to tire easily and limited how long he could focus on tasks. Her explanation of how short-term memory loss affected his ability to plan and achieve even simple tasks was simple but informative.

"With continuous repetition of the same routine, short-term memory becomes mid-term memory, and then hopefully long-term memory. Stimulating the right side of the brain in a consistent and repetitive manner can open up new pathways and reroute damaged neurons. The brain can repair itself, but it takes consistent approaches and time."

Wendy believed it was important for everyone to know who Bill had been, and still was.

"This was a highly intelligent man with a great sense of humour and a truly loving and kind spirit. But now he responds to Catherine's stresses instinctively, and it's not good for him. Consistency is imperative for success. His lack of awareness of his limitations, like walking, is good news because he keeps working on his programs. But that means you can't let him out of your sight. This is why it is so important that he has the right, and the same, people consistently. This would provide true continuity and would be far, far less stressful for both Bill and Catherine. Ultimately, we all want the best for Bill."

Jan expressed why she felt it was essential to have the same nurse to do evening meds, catheter, and other evening care.

"It puts Bill in jeopardy every time a new nurse arrives who can't use the lift or other equipment."

Everyone had an opportunity to ask questions, clarify areas of concern, and make suggestions. With the issues seemingly well understood by all, we disbanded.

"Finally there is hope!" I thought.

But just as Wendy was going out the door, the nursing agency supervisor stopped, turned to me, and said, "I still don't see why he needs the same people. If he has no short-term memory, he won't remember who was here yesterday."

I was dumbfounded.

However, thanks to Wendy's meeting, the scheduling did improve. Jan had become an expert on Bill, and did most of the orientation with Susan, which was a relief for me. Jan's knowledge of brain issues was a major contribution to Susan, and her knowledge of medical issues was a major contribution to Jan. Bill benefitted greatly, and his interactions with each of them continued to be very positive.

Kevin continued to be a regular, too, referring to his visits as "Tuesdays with Bill," a play on the title of a currently popular book. They had come so far together. The two of them made good use of the kids' basketball stand I had scored at a thrift store and challenged each other to playoffs regularly. The ceiling pulleys became a pulling apparatus, which from upstairs sounded like they were using a bucksaw.

Jeopardy became a contest between them, too. Bill was talking so much more to his new friend now. Kevin's persistence was paying off. It was heart-warming to see Bill interacting with another guy who was just a buddy, one who had no expectations. Fun, companionship, and joy showed on both of their faces.

CHRISTMAS 2004 WAS quickly approaching. Decorating the house was still an important tradition. Although Bill couldn't stand up to hang the decorations on the tree, he could do it from his chair. He was much more engaged in the whole event than the year before.

My sister, Brenda, showed Bill a project she had found in a magazine. He liked the idea — painting snow scenes on large galvanized buckets — and they agreed they should make several together. I shopped for the materials, but otherwise took no part in the creativity, except for sneaking in with the video camera.

I was enthralled as I watched them in action. Bill followed Brenda's directions, periodically quipping about the personalities of the snowmen. They chatted about which bucket would be for which friend. What colours did he want to use? How would they wrap them? Blue sky, white snow, and a large snowman, complete with orange carrot-like nose and Bill's signature, completed the artwork. Then they filled each bucket with driveway salt and a scoop.

The pride Bill took in creating those treasures was evident, and I was touched watching my sister help him with something that was so good for his spirit.

We had lots of visitors, both close friends and family, over the season, and Bill was proud to present his salt buckets to their recipients. Kevin was almost tearful at the sight of his salt bucket and even more touched by the card Bill had chosen for him: "To My Special Friend."

One of my favourite memories of that holiday is of Kevin's narration of a special outing with Bill. After touring the Christmas Lights Festival at a nearby park, the two men decided to go to Tim Hortons for a hot drink and food. Bill ordered beef stew, milk, and a maple donut. Partway through the meal, he began spooning the stew onto the donut as if it were crusty bread. Kevin made mention of this oddity to Bill.

"It's really, really good this way," Bill said.

To each his own.

Another high point was Christmas dinner at Earl and Joyce's home. Our local wheelchair transport company had a woman on staff who always worked Christmas Day to ensure that disabled people were not shut-ins. This wonderful woman delivered us (and a salt bucket) to our destination with as much delight as I felt. Being out at such a special event, with such good friends, had been a long time coming. Yes, Virginia, there is a Santa Claus.

Listening to holiday music, enjoying our tree together, and sharing our home and very different life with family and friends all contributed to a joyous season. It had been quite a year.

PART FOUR

REHABILITATION, TOGETHER

30

PAINTING LESSONS

THE NEW YEAR, 2005, arrived. The holidays had been remarkable, but alas, all good things must end. We needed to get back to the business of rehabilitation. Together.

From Wendy I learned about Conductive Education, a program established in Europe during World War II. Its purpose was to maximize the functionality of children with neurological problems. Since being introduced in North America, it was being widely used for adult advancement as well. The program was very expensive, but I believed we'd gain much from it.

For the first session Bill and I went alone. Sydney, who was the "conductor," and her assistant helped us into the therapy room and got right down to work.

They used wooden slatted benches, about four feet wide and over six feet long. They looked mighty uncomfortable. Sydney explained that when you can feel discomfort, you can learn to feel where your muscles and bones are, and then adjust. She worked at getting Bill to use the wall bars to try pulling himself up out of the chair, explaining how this uses the brain, the whole body, and speech. She encouraged Bill to keep saying, with each movement, "Reaching, sitting tall, reaching, and sitting back again."

Next she had Bill lie on his back on a platform and do a variety of exercises with her, some for range of motion, some for improving hand–eye coordination, and some just for stretching and breathing. With each movement she asked him to repeat, three times: "I push my left leg out, I push my left leg out, I push my left leg out, out, out, out."

I was delighted to see him doing as she asked, and so quickly. I mused, as I watched, that even though Bill didn't fully understand this program, it seemed worthwhile to him, so he was participating. Things that were pointless to him got very little of his attention. Our session seemed to fly by, but I'd seen so much and gotten so many new ideas, I was anxious to get to work on them at home.

Our next two sessions were similar: repeating the same motions and phrases. Sometimes Bill participated in the whole exercise; sometimes he did the motions but not the speech; but each day was encouraging and educational. I was delighted that Wendy and Jan joined us for the last session: Wendy because she had recommended it, Jan because she would be the one to follow through with the program at home when I was at work.

Their eyes lit up when Bill wheeled over to the wall bars and demonstrated his pull-ups. They both understood how this could be key to getting him back on his feet. They also understood the value of the overall muscle work it involved. Bill was enjoying showing off for them. The high point was when, at the end of the session, he said goodbye to Sydney, then looked directly into the video camera, waved, and signed out with, "Goodbye for now."

WENDY, STILL SERVING as coach, teacher, guide, and often confidante, continued to support and encourage us. Through her agency she brought us someone new, David, a mature student in his early thirties, to do a co-op placement with Bill.

She and I had often talked about how good it would be for Bill to have more interaction with men. By now, old friends seemed scarce. In my kinder moods I tried to remind myself it was very hard for them to see Bill with such disabilities.

Then I'd rage to myself, "Bullshit! This is no picnic for him. They would be getting the easier part. They might be uncomfortable, but he's fighting for his very existence, and friends would be like manna from heaven. Those who knew him before his brain injury would still have been able to talk to him about old times."

I was hurt, for him, but I realized it wasn't going to change. This made the prospect of a new guy working with him more intriguing. Bill, as usual, was agreeable.

As the weeks went by, and they accomplished much together, David proposed a new option. He was an artist and volunteered to give Bill painting lessons.

When his co-op period was finished, the teacher and student began their first lesson. I watched from the stairwell the first time David set up his easel and painting supplies. Bill looked at the blank canvas with an equally blank look. Then his expression changed. Something remembered? Did he think this was a test? Did David think he was a painter? David calmly explained the first step.

"You cover the whole white canvas with a white primer, Bill."

"Why would I cover something white with more white?"

A logical response, I thought. Bill had a very practical mind. For many minutes he just watched the primer being applied, and explained, by his new teacher. Alternately, he would pick up a brush or a paint knife and examine it intently, studying every detail, even reading the brand name aloud.

If David asked a question, he might or might not get a response, which was something he had already experienced during his co-op time. Bill's silence would continue at times throughout their new lessons, but less frequently.

Sometimes, Bill made a tremendous effort to duplicate a particular brush stroke his teacher demonstrated. But often he branched out with his own "technique." Other times, David did everything but stand on his head to get Bill to participate, to no avail. The student would become a statue. Often in these lessons Bill chatted amiably with his art teacher, expressing interest in the project. Other times he retreated into his own private place. This was a world even I couldn't get into.

I was deeply touched by the patience and support David accorded his novice student. On a bad day, he proceeded with the lesson as if his protégé were actively participating, hoping it would happen, and often Bill suddenly took part. The younger man was always respectful of Bill's sense of himself. Together they discovered Bill had a talent for using the sculpting knife to add depth and texture to mountain peaks.

This brought rave reviews from the teacher. It brought a river of tears from me.

Their first work of art, which took months to complete, had begun with no fixed plan and meandered through many phases and changes. When it was finished, both artists put their initials on it, David using the hand-over-hand approach to help Bill form the letters.

I immediately took it for framing and hung it over our fireplace, in full view of all who crossed our threshold. I revelled in the pride Bill displayed each time someone saw it for the first time. I loved it when he would direct a cheeky grin at me and then act as though he had been turning out acrylic paintings forever. What a ham.

I was surprised again by how many things I didn't know about his childhood when one of his older brothers told me about the art contest Bill had won in school. He had reproduced the Cape Breton landscape out the window of his schoolroom and won a prize for it, a book he had treasured for years. I asked Bill why he had never told me about this particular honour.

"I can't remember everything!" he said. "Besides, then there would be no mystery about me any more."

Brain injury, my ass! This man would always find ways to make me laugh.

IN EARLY MARCH, when I called Frank, the physiotherapist, his office manager said he was still at the pool.

"At the pool? The *pool?*" I thought.

I had long considered that weight-bearing exercises would be safer, easier, and certainly more fun for Bill in a pool. Having grown up by the ocean, he loved the water. I had unsuccessfully tried the previous year to find someone willing to try pool work with him. The home care physiotherapists are not allowed to provide services outside the patient's home. Private therapists in our area didn't do house calls or pool work.

I was ecstatic when Frank said, "I never even thought about this for Bill, but I'm certainly willing to give it a try."

The closest pool with a hydraulic chairlift was at the Belleville School for the Deaf, twenty kilometres from home, but the local wheelchair-accessible van service could accommodate us at a mere twenty dollars for the round trip. We made the arrangements and reorganized Bill's schedule to incorporate this new opportunity. I was disappointed that Friday was to be the first day because I couldn't take another day off work. Susan took on the task with great enthusiasm, though. It was unnerving to send Bill out into the world without me, but it was a golden opportunity, and I trusted Frank and the nurse completely. Our friend Earl volunteered to videotape the session so at least I could see it when I got home. Late in the afternoon Susan phoned to tell me the venture had been a great success.

Once home I rushed to start the video. Bill and Jan formed up the rest of the audience.

The video opened with Bill by the pool sitting on a chair that looked much like his shower chair. Frank hauled Bill up out of the chair, pivoted, and plopped him down on the hydraulic chair lift and belted him in. I chuckled hearing Bill's very loud, very exaggerated groan. As the process continued Bill looked a little startled but nothing more. Susan began turning the lift chair, while Frank slithered into the pool. Within half a minute the chair had been lowered, Bill was in the water, and he had floated off the chair. He looked incredulous. He was free!

Susan and Frank positioned themselves on either side of Bill. Frank was watching him for any signs of a problem, and said, "Bill, try to put your feet on the bottom and your hands on the pool edge." Susan cheered as he accomplished the feat.

"Try to stretch up and down now, Bill," Frank said in a companionable tone. "Again. And again."

Bill was bobbing away, and Susan was congratulating him.

"Try to lean back and just relax, Bill," Frank said.

Bill wasn't as quick to try that, or so it appeared. I could see they didn't realize he was trying to keep his hair dry. Vanity, thy name is…man. Finally he did relax and started to float on his back. When asked, he put his feet and legs up. Frank braced against them with his hands and body weight. Right on cue, Bill pushed against Frank with all his might. He was propelled backward to Susan, who gave him a little push back to Frank. All three laughed as they repeated the process a dozen times.

"I feel like the monkey in the middle," Bill said.

Before they turned him loose again, Frank showed him how to walk sideways along the pool length, holding onto the sides of the pool, crossing his feet over in a crab crawl. He demonstrated how he could push himself up to a standing position.

I watched Bill follow the instructions. Up and down, up and down, up and down he bobbed.

Occasionally Bill looked like he was ignoring them. I could tell he was listening intently to a conversation in another area of the pool as he gazed around, taking in other details of the pool and all the different people.

He was getting really good at bobbing up and down. Susan encouraged him and even gave him a little competition, showing him how high she could go. He tried even harder, determined to do his best for these two.

It jolted me to see Bill heading to the deep end. Frank brought him back, but almost immediately he headed for the deep again. Frank brought him back again. They repeated this a few times. Bill had never had any fear of water, and today he seemed oblivious to needing Frank's help.

Then I watched Bill head to the middle of the pool with Frank. It didn't appear any deeper there, but there was nothing to hold onto. I could see his arms and legs moving to tread water. Then, quickly, Frank's hands were up in the air. He was definitely sending *me* the message, "Bill has absolutely no support from me."

Watching the video was *almost* as good as being there. Bill was also watching himself on the screen. He was grinning, and sometimes smirking. Pointing to the screen, he said, "Look at the whale."

I squinted to see what he meant. There, behind him, was a very, very large person jumping around doing exercises. Although it made me laugh, I hoped he hadn't said it then, out loud.

There was another round of Bill pushing off the side of the pool with his legs. I saw his limbs stretching out farther. He was putting a lot of strength and energy into those pushes, trying to knock Frank off balance. When Bill suddenly took in a great gulp of water and started coughing, Susan and Frank laughed at him instead of panicking.

Next it was time to do the extraction procedure. Reversing the entry process went seamlessly, although it appeared to bewilder Bill, who asked, "Why can't I just climb out myself?" Once again I recognized his limited perception of his disabilities.

When the video ended, with Bill flashing a final smile and waving at the camera, I had to leave Bill and Jan for a few minutes. I bolted upstairs to our old bedroom for a cry, but it felt wonderful to be crying over something so very positive for a change.

31

A REAL SHOCKER

Of course, by Monday there was an agency problem.

"The nurse isn't allowed to do any of this," I was told. "She isn't to leave your home during her shift."

I would have understood her not being allowed to go in the pool alone with Bill, but an experienced therapist was present who assumed all the responsibilities. Couldn't she at least travel with him and watch him? Damn. It seemed Bill couldn't have anything go well without a rules problem coming up.

Many phone calls, different interpretations, and much checking with the higher-ups eventually resulted in the decision that Susan could go *to* the pool with Bill, but not *into* it. At least that was far better than not being allowed to take him at all.

We decided Bill and I would go to the pool on Mondays and Wednesdays, and Susan would go on Fridays. Every week we saw a stronger, happier Bill. This lightened my spirits immensely.

Although it required extra effort to get ready to go, and an earlier start to the day, Bill loved his newfound freedom, and I loved it for him. We continued with the swimming therapy until the end of June, when suddenly the school decided to close the pool to the public.

I WAS ENCOURAGED by Bill's progress, his spirit, and his determination, but I often travelled in and out of a bleak place emotionally. I was still angry and frustrated that he had been denied opportunities for rehab. I had coined a phrase about myself, which I shared with no one: "schizofrantic." One hour I was elated and optimistic; the next hour I was engulfed in anxiety and fear, struggling to contain my worries about our circumstances.

One day in late March while I was at work, I was feeling particularly low. It wasn't about Bill, though. It was about work, money, and energy. My career was suffering seriously. Not being back to work full-time was weighing on me and costing me dearly, in clients, income, and my sense of balance. My creativity had been all but extinguished. Success at work had always been a big part of my sense of self, and now the energy it was taking to wear so many hats was telling on me. I nearly always felt I was failing in one realm or another.

The additional concerns and the frustrations of always being in "training mode" with new home care people depleted my energy and patience. I resented how much time it took away from Bill and me. I was slipping back into the abyss. There were even times when I found myself being impatient with Bill. I was in a constant state of sleep deprivation. There were hundreds of small things I was trying to keep track of. Sometimes it was hard for me to focus on what we had already achieved. I rarely gave in to feeling sorry for us, but this day, I seemed to be giving it free rein.

Then I received a phone call. In an appointment-based business, the phone ringing was essential. But each time it did, I had a mini-panic attack, always expecting something was wrong at home. And often, it was. This call, however, was very different.

Terri, from the Chedoke rehab centre, was on the line to ask me if I could use some extra help. Financial help.

I laughed and said, "I was trying to decide earlier which I needed most: a secretary, a slave, or a financial benefactor. Any one of those would be helpful."

She said some funding was being allocated for Bill, and someone would be arranging a meeting with us soon. It sounded like a miracle. I had already learned that miracles often came our way when I was at my lowest point emotionally.

A week later, at the beginning of April, I attended that meeting. Wendy had told me there might be as much as six hundred and fifty dollars a month allocated to help Bill. Finally we might be able to afford the private physiotherapist who had brought Bill so far already. It would certainly help me manage our costs more easily. Maybe at last we could finance that amazing standing frame. I was cautiously optimistic that this was an answer to my prayers.

Asked to provide receipts for some of our expenditures, I had riffled through my growing stack of bills, paid and unpaid. I arrived at the Regional Community Brain Injury Services office in Belleville full of mixed feelings, reminding myself not to get too hopeful. The thought of the extra money per month overwhelmed me. But what if Wendy had misunderstood?

In the conference room I met Wendy, Dr. Carlson, Dawn (the director of RCBIS), and several other staff. When they announced, "We are giving you and Bill a one-time-only cheque for sixty-five hundred dollars," I was relieved beyond words.

THEN CAME THE REAL shocker: The Ministry of Health had allocated special individualized funding to Bill — seventy-eight thousand dollars a year.

"This must be a dream. This isn't really happening, is it?" I whispered to Wendy, trying to remain calm.

Part of the money would fund a real rehabilitation counsellor.

Professional rehab was now within Bill's grasp. Finally, he would have the opportunity he had been denied for so long. The money would not come to us directly, but would be distributed through the agency. I was relieved, as I had enough money issues to deal with. I didn't want more.

I left that meeting floating. How had this magic come into our life to finally give us the help we needed? I realized we were about to be saved: Bill would finally get proper professional help, and I would be able to go back to work full-time. It would take some time to put this funding in place, but it would be soon.

Hallelujah! Life was once again on the upswing for Bill and me.

32

WHERE THE REHAB IS

On may 4, 2005, it was time to deliver on a promise. Months earlier, Wendy had asked if I would speak at a conference in Hamilton for professionals in the brain injury realm, including doctors, nurses, physio and occupational therapists, speech and recreational therapists, and case managers. I said yes, reluctantly because I felt an obligation to her and her office, and, despite my anger and frustration with the system, I still believed many people were doing the best they could to help us.

And I had an ulterior motive. I wanted, no, I needed, to show that our amateur home rehabilitation program was working. I needed our story to make a difference. I needed to show these people what the health care system had expected us to give up. Our life together. They needed to see what we were doing, and to realize it was a viable option, not just for us but perhaps for many others. The established thinking had to be changed.

I had a guilty little secret, too: I was looking forward to a night in a luxury hotel, and a night in which I wouldn't be waking hourly to reassure myself that my husband was still breathing. After checking in at the Sheraton and enjoying a lovely meal, complete with fine wine, I was content to retire to my room and total privacy. A long soak in the bath, followed by a longer read of a new book, added to the luxurious feeling.

At ten o'clock the next morning, Wendy and I attended a presentation by Dr. Carlson about his research study proving the theory that "it is better to do to learn than learn to do." As he spoke, I thought about how much value Bill and I would have gotten from this study. Even a short period of real rehab, early on, and the use of equipment like a standing frame to build up his muscles, balance, and strength would have been invaluable.

It had become clear to me long before that it wasn't his ability to stand that Bill had lost, but his strength and balance from all those months in bed. The doctor's evidence-based study contained solid data. The most significant information I gleaned was that brain injury recovery was possible for a much longer period than previously believed, up to ten years and more. Much of the information was beyond my scope, but the audience of professionals was enthralled. This study could significantly influence changes in the methods and funding of brain injury rehab.

The second presentation was by a woman telling her son's story. At seventeen, he had been the victim of a brutal, unprovoked attack by violent strangers. His injuries were life threatening. He sustained a severe brain injury. Life and death hung in the balance for many, many days.

To her credit, and my amazement, the attack was not her focus. Instead, she was intent on giving credit to the professionals. The Hamilton area has significant acquired brain injury programs, and her family was, according to her, fortunate to live in that region.

With a very professional and colourful slide show she described her son's journey immediately following surgery. The slides demonstrated the great patience and dedication of the therapists in the acute care hospital. Once her son was medically stable, several months later, he was moved to a private facility dedicated exclusively to brain injury rehabilitation.

Although his potential for progress was still very much unknown, the staff were dedicated to giving him the best possible therapies. Pictures appeared on the screen showing two and three therapists physically supporting him as he took his first step since the attack. Speech therapists were diligent in working through his various voice projection and swallowing problems.

"Our entire family was embraced and included in our son's therapy," she told the audience. "We received an incredible education in the many ways we, too, could help him. Learning to understand the multitude of brain-related problems he would have to struggle with, likely for the rest of his life, and how we could help him cope, kept us from ever feeling sorry for him. Or us. He will not likely ever live independently again, but we have learned to take one step at a time."

My mind darted away for a moment. "How did he get such amazing help? Did this come from the same health care system I've been battling with for so long?"

The mother reclaimed my attention when she clicked a new picture onto the screen. After nearly two years in specialized rehab, her son was making his first visit home. He was pictured standing between his two brothers, who were supporting him, grinning into the camera.

A choking sensation overtook me. I had to escape. I fled to the empty hallway. Tears pooled. Anger bubbled up like a new oil strike. I was sweating and my heart was racing. I gulped in air as fast as I could, fighting the urge to scream.

Questions ricocheted around in my mind. "Why was our story so different from theirs? Who decides who gets what help? Who decides which patients are more likely to be a success story? Was it age? Why would the medical system think Bill, at fifty-six, was disposable? This young man's early prognosis didn't sound any more optimistic or hopeful than Bill's."

Walter Gretzky's book floated through my memory. He, too, had received an amazing rehabilitation and recovery program. I was shocked by my own jealousy. How could I be jealous of this woman and her son's experience? How could I be jealous of Mr. Gretzky, and his family, and the progress he had made?

I waited in a cool, hidden alcove for the session to end and for Wendy to emerge. It had taken me every second of ten minutes to calm down and think clearly again. I knew from her expression she understood what had happened to me in that lecture hall.

"This is most likely insurance money or a very large legal settlement, Catherine."

"I didn't know what an enormous difference money, settlements, and disability or critical illness insurance could make," was my regret-filled response.

A large ballroom was set for lunch. We found our seats at a table with Dr. Carlson and several other people from their circle. This was no average lunch. It was a five-star hotel lunch. Wendy enlightened me about the conference as we ate.

"This entire conference — the meals, the drinks, the 'nightclub' down the hall where sushi can be had at the end of the day — is all paid for by private firms. Law firms. Accounting firms. These firms will be competing for the business of managing and representing brain injury people with insurance settlements. Big settlements. This is how and where they romance the case managers."

The lunch chatter brought me back to earth emotionally, and I was able to regroup by the time dessert was served.

MY PRESENTATION WAS titled "Home Is Where the Heart and Rehabilitation Is." Wendy first introduced herself and her agency and spoke of their services in eastern Ontario. She spoke of the unique issues and needs there. She briefly explained how she had come to meet Bill and me, and what insights her experiences with us had yielded. She bragged, on our behalf, about what we had been able to overcome together.

Then she introduced me. I was quaking inside as I crossed to centre stage, but as soon as I started to speak, the words flowed easily. I told the audience some of Bill's history that led to the nursing home recommendation. I told them a little about us, and our life pre-brain injury, and why being together was so important for both of us — and how deadly and devastating life in a nursing home would have been.

"From the first weeks following Bill's complications, I became very aware of the negativity of most of the professionals who dealt with us. Their close-mindedness shocked me, and its psychological damage was monumental to both of us. No one seemed to think Bill could progress. The specific reasons remain unclear to me, but I believe that lack of communication, on every level, was a very important factor. Incorrect assumptions have run rampant through our journey. Many of the professionals assumed I was just a wife in denial. Going home turned out to be the best, and safest, thing for us to do."

I had put together a very amateur twenty-minute video of what I considered to be the most valuable parts of our life together. I wanted this audience to know the face of the person this story belonged to. A few minutes of history, in still photos, showed Bill as a very young soldier, a handsome groom, an adoring uncle, a man with nine caring siblings, a man who adored his furry little dog. And showed a man and a woman who loved each other completely.

I pressed the pause button.

"My husband was a very independent and determined man. He still is, although independent is a relative term in our house now. When Bill came home in July of 2003, he was enormously de-conditioned. He struggled to remain awake for more than an hour or two, had difficulty carrying out the most basic tasks of everyday life: shaving, brushing his teeth, sitting up. As we crept along, developing a routine to help him regain lost skills, mostly by guesswork and by God, he made huge advances.

"My struggles to find home care staff who were rehab-minded have been endless. Those who are dedicated to helping Bill have been such a blessing, but I am still angry with a system that gave up on him so early, four weeks into his post-surgery complications. Being declared 'disposable' was a devastating blow. Early intervention, any intervention for that matter, would have made a vast difference in our journey."

I paused to catch my breath and stay calm.

"Competent home care staff with rehabilitation skills were a rarity in our home. Continuity was incredibly difficult to maintain. I did not have a clue what the financial issues of this would be. Good thing I didn't. I never realized that two and a half years later I still wouldn't be back to work full-time. There were a thousand things I didn't know, including that we would sink into an ocean of debt, but I did know we would do anything for each other, and we would make a new life. I bet some of you are thinking I need anger management counselling."

Most of the audience laughed, but I sensed they realized how serious this was.

"The other thing I didn't know, until this morning, was the value of insurance and legal settlements. Had I known, just before I dialled 911, I could have backed over Bill with the car and he could have sued me."

This time the audience didn't laugh.

"Knowing that a nursing home was the only solution offered by the hospitals and our health care system, I want you to see some pieces of his life now. Our life."

I pressed the play button again and watched with the audience as Bill appeared on the screen.

He was totally focused on the miniature hockey game on the table. With shot after shot he sent the puck flying down into Kevin's end. When he scored, the tiny rink played a tune, like a lottery kiosk. Bill grinned at Kevin and said, "Gotcha!"

The next scene showed Bill at the punching bag. He used a left hook, then a right jab to send it reeling. He punched right-handed, left-handed, then with both hands.

Off camera, Michele was saying, "Okay, Bill, now do three right-handed, three left-handed, and three punches with both hands."

His posture was perfect. He followed her instructions until both hands were required. He stopped. Putting both hands on the bright red punching bag, he pulled it close and examined every seam, every letter printed on the side, and even put his ear against it, listening to who knew what?

Another scene began. Bill was in the middle of a swimming pool using only a Styrofoam noodle for support. He was alternately dog paddling and treading water. Grinning at Frank, he shot a splash of water at the therapist.

Next, he was sitting at the easel, studying the brush in his hand. In a flurry, he brushed green acrylic paint on the canvas, the brush strokes smooth, rhythmic, gentle. He brushed outward, softening the green until the grass looked shrouded in mist. David, the art teacher, was mesmerized. It was beautiful.

Next he was sitting in his wheelchair beside the bed, folding his laundry, carefully smoothing out any unwanted wrinkles and creases. Then he was sitting at the table, carefully forming the pastry for turnovers around blueberry filling. He examined each item carefully, then declared, "Ready for the oven."

The video ran for ten minutes more, showing six or seven of his everyday activities: dinner with family on the back porch, opening presents on Christmas morning, throwing toys for his puppy, shaving, brushing his hair, and watching a golf tournament, complete with his own commentary. I pushed the pause button again.

"Imagine how much more might have been possible," I said. "Imagine how much more might already have been accomplished. Imagine what you would want for your own husband, wife, child. Do any of you think, as I do, that Bill deserved better than to spend the rest of his life in a nursing home?"

I pushed the play button for the last time, saying, "This is the greatest reason life at home is better for us than a nursing home institution."

There we were, propped up in bed, shoulder to shoulder, drinking our coffee, watching the morning news. Jessie was clambering over me to get her treats from Bill. In the background, a CD played the words of Shania Twain's song "You're Still the One," with its now immortal (to us) lines:

They said "I bet they'll never make it"
But just look at us holding on,
We're still together, still going strong.

Along with lines about beating the odds together:

I'm glad we didn't listen,
Look at what we would be missing.

As I turned off the video, I could see many tear-streaked faces. They understood. Quietly, I said, "As you continue in your work, please remember: Where there's a will, there may very well be a way. Please be inspired by Bill, by love, by commitment, by desperation. Please remember us."

33

FARTHER DOWN
THE RABBIT HOLE

Summer 2005 breezed in gently, still with undulating hills and valleys, but without the mountains and craters of the previous year. Bill had been without any serious medical problems or complications for a long stretch, and he was improving in so many realms. He was doing very, very well. All things considered.

But all was not well with me. Two and a half years had passed since this journey began, and I missed our former life far more than I would acknowledge. My deep sadness, grief, and depression were things I could not share with anyone. Friends who had been our nucleus for years, some close, some casual, had all but vanished. Had I alienated them, perhaps even made them feel unwelcome? Catapulting from one crisis to another absorbed so much of my time and energy. Learning what I needed to know to make our new life work compelled me. My fury at the system that had so completely let us down consumed me.

"If there's anything we can do, let us know," now seemed like an empty, shallow offer, and I didn't know how to ask for what we needed most: anything that brought normal back into our life. Visiting Bill to let him know he still mattered to them; running errands to give me a break; easy meals I wouldn't have to prepare; assuring us that we were still two living, breathing people. Come to see us, but please don't treat us differently, please do not judge.

This loss was manifesting itself as sadness and anger and disappointment. And I was devastated for Bill's loss. I made a mental note to myself. "Once we have our heads above water again, I will be a better friend to everyone who matters to me."

My sister, Brenda, was still living with us. We had never experienced any tension growing up — she being ten years older than I — and at first her residence with us was helpful. However, the intensity of the fight that Bill and I were waging for our life together was a different matter. Brenda and I frequently had little, and not so little, squabbles. The helpful hints from Big Sister often were the polar opposite of how I wanted to do things. Unable to ignore these intrusions, well intentioned though they were, I would launch a counter-attack. Yelling matches erupted. We hurt each other often, and often deeply.

It so often felt like the Freight Train of Unsolicited Opinions and Advice roared into my life from other places, too. So many people, professionals and amateurs alike, believed they knew more, and knew better, about Bill than I did. In some instances they were right, but after so many miscommunications and disagreements I usually ended up just feeling wounded.

I even had mixed feelings about the infringements on our space, companionship, and privacy. It no longer mattered who it was. It only mattered that it was. Home care nurses, personal support workers, the skin nurse, the occupational therapist, the speech therapist, Frank, equipment people, even those I liked and appreciated, often felt like invaders. For most of these people, this was their place of work. For us, it was our home, our fortress. Precious little of it was really ours now. Privacy, which had always been so important to both of us, no longer existed.

My reactions to my sister, and many others, were arguably extreme. I thought I was just overtired. As I experienced the ups and downs and confusion about our lost life, I kept everything locked inside. I was afraid any complaint would sound as though I didn't want to do this any more, or that I couldn't cope. I had rarely shared private concerns with anyone but Bill. But these issues I could not share with him, either, which gave them extra weight.

Finally, and very reluctantly, I accepted the case manager's suggestion that I talk to the Home Care social worker. Fearful of sounding like a frantic lunatic, I tried to articulate my specific and practical concerns and fears.

"You have to understand, my fears are not so much about coping with Bill's circumstances or his rehabilitation. If money were no object, this would only be one-tenth as hard as it is right now. I really believed I would be back to work full-time ages ago, and it feels like I've been struggling over money forever. The solution is getting back to work full-time, but I can't do that. I certainly can't leave Bill alone, and the health care system is already giving him significantly more coverage than normal."

I paused to calm myself down.

"The special funding they said was allocated five months ago hasn't come through. I feel as though my only serious options today are to sell our home, give up our dog, move to an apartment, figure out how Bill will shower or bathe and still make progress, *or* take Bill and Jessie into the garage with me, start the car, and wait for carbon monoxide to end my worries." Seeing her raised eyebrows I quickly added, "Of course I am not going to do that, but it frightens me that it would even cross my mind."

She listened intently to my diatribe, but beyond providing me with a sounding board and giving me few placating comments, she had no practical suggestions to offer.

"I wish I could be of more help," she said, "but anytime you need to talk, I'm always available."

Later, the case manager asked me: "Was it cathartic or helpful to be able to talk, in confidence, with her?"

No. In fact, it made it worse. In my mind she was just another well-paid but ineffective part of the system. I found myself farther down the rabbit hole, sinking in negatives.

KEVIN WAS A constant, though. Most Tuesday evenings he and Bill still visited on the back deck, often breaking into a game of catch or "make Kevin chase things." Sometimes Al, our neighbour, came out to the fence to see Jessie and talk to Bill.

Al usually waved and said, "Hi, Bill, how are you?"

Bill would wave and say, "Hi, Al, I'm good."

"Nice day, isn't it?"

"Sure is!"

"Are you beating Kevin at lawn darts?"

"Sure am!"

Just a normal chat with a neighbour.

Bill still had significant initiation issues, though, and it was difficult for him to start a conversation. He most always responded, and usually correctly, to questions, but the asker had to wait patiently for the response. It's a difficult concept for people to grasp. Many of the home care workers still didn't understand, but then it just wasn't part of their training. Frequently, one of them would ask Bill a question, then immediately answer it, like a very poor interviewer. It disturbed me that so few realized how detrimental this could be. Did they think he was an imbecile?

I appreciated the pauses in his exchanges with Kevin, who waited up to thirty seconds for an answer to his question before he asked again. If he still got no response. He changed the question or answered it as an anecdote to entertain Bill. The two friends frequently rolled around the neighbourhood, discussing the various trucks and cars they saw, the state of people's grass, and military people in the area they both knew. Sometimes I heard them coming down the street, chatting amiably about the flowers and birds. That lightened my spirit, at least temporarily. And by now even temporary respite was invaluable.

34

THE CAVALRY ALMOST ARRIVED

AND THEN, IN JUNE of that year, the seizure issue reared its ugly head again.

What I had learned along the way about how the system works paid off, though. There was no delay in getting him admitted to Kingston General and under the care of a neurologist this time. Bill spent a week there being monitored by Dr. Spiller. Tracking these seizures to another urinary tract infection, she was able to contain Bill's hospital stay to a relatively simple experience. This time, while she adjusted medications and ran various tests, we had what amounted to a mini-holiday. Bill was fairly well, so we played ball, read magazines, curled up on the bed together, and went to the café often for treats.

It still disturbed me that Bill lived his life enduring three catheter insertions a day, which were often the cause of these infections, and I wondered whether he'd be dealing with these problems today if the catheter been removed much sooner, back in the winter of 2003.

TOWARD THE END of July, Wendy's agency, which would manage the special funding, had recommended a full-time rehabilitation counsellor. But until written authorization from the Ministry of Health arrived, we just had to wait. The agency hadn't yet received the paperwork and wasn't going to risk having its budget negatively impacted.

It was difficult for me to keep from venting my frustration about the delay on Wendy, or anyone else for that matter. I seemed to always be asking the same questions.

"But the ministry has confirmed that this funding will be available! How much longer does Bill have to wait for help? How much more buried in debt do I have to get? I was first told about this in March. We've been waiting for the cavalry for more than four months. Why does everything take so long? Doesn't anyone else realize that Bill's window of opportunity is shrinking daily?"

Wendy encouraged me to focus on how to best utilize the funding to help Bill. She told me her agency had recommended that a full-time rehab counsellor be hired to do what I was doing with Bill now.

"You can finally go back to work full-time. How does that sound?"

It sounded incredible, but I was only cautiously optimistic.

Wendy and I agreed that Jan was the perfect choice for this new position. She was qualified and had prior experience with the agency. Already up to speed about Bill's health issues, she could do the toileting, skin care, and the transfers, and she would put her heart and soul into the job. Most importantly, Bill and I trusted her completely.

Finally, on August 20, I was informed that the authorization from the Ministry of Health for the funding was secured. Now Bill would finally get the help he needed to move farther forward. I'd talked so much about the enormous value of getting Bill more physio with Frank. Would Bill finally be able to get a standing frame? Perhaps the transportation costs and pool membership wouldn't be so hard to cover now. Now it would be possible to get him some other creative outlets. This would be the most amazing breakthrough point, for both of us. What had been only glimmers of possibility now would become realities. The cavalry had finally arrived.

Well, not exactly.

Wendy's next unpleasant task was to explain to me how the process worked (or didn't, depending on your perspective). "Jan can't be hired just because you want her. It's a union job, so it has to be posted at our various offices first. If no one applies it will be posted 'out' and Jan can apply. She'll be a shoo-in. After all, she's already doing the job *and* supporting the training of home care staff."

"It all sounds like just more of the same — bureaucracy, red tape and union b.s.," I said. "But, as long as the outcome is in Bill's best interest, I don't care how they get to it. I just want them to hurry up and get there."

Then, a few days later, the bombshell. Wendy had to tell me that someone, only one person, did apply in-office and had been hired.

"But with only one applicant, how do they know this is the best person?" I asked. "Do they have a job description for a day with Bill MacLeod? Shouldn't she at least have to meet us? Doesn't she even have to meet Bill and demonstrate that she *can* do the job? Is that even part of the equation?"

"Union rules, Catherine."

Another journey through bureaucracy.

Although I argued against the decision to hire this candidate, another stranger, fearing it would take me another enormous amount of time and energy to train someone else, my opinion carried no weight. Jan was capable and current. Bill liked her, was secure with her, and worked hard with her. He was flourishing with her. Why should either of us be forced accept a new face and new approaches?

Wendy asked the agency to reconsider. The answer: "This is the procedure. Union rules must be adhered to."

I prayed fervently that the new counsellor would be as skilled, as competent, and just as able to connect with Bill as Jan.

Bile rose up in my throat when I imagined another new person in Bill's life: further erosion of his dignity, and greater risk of setbacks and mistakes. But, realizing that arguing was futile, I buried my outrage and accepted their choice. I needed to move on. I explained to Bill he would soon have his own assistant.

"She'll be your new life coach, help you to make even more progress, and get me out of your face."

He grinned, seeming keen on that last part.

When Colleen, also a graduate of Behavioural Sciences, came to meet us during the week that followed the meeting, she seemed bright and friendly and included Bill in the discussion. She recited her group home experience.

"I usually spend an hour or two every week helping our clients do things like balancing their chequebooks, going grocery shopping with them, organizing their rooms, and doing other practical stuff."

I realized something was amiss, and asked her, "Have you ever worked with a person in their own home like our situation?"

"Well, no. Only with people in group homes."

"Have you ever worked with physio equipment or done pivot transfers?"

"Well, no."

"Have you ever done toileting routines with a person in a wheelchair? Or physio work?"

"Well, no."

She might have an academic education in brain injury and cognitive issues, but what the hell had she done that qualified her for this job? I tried to find some good in this. At least she could learn the rest, if Bill and I still had the endurance to teach it, again. Wendy and I ironed out a plan to maximize the value of Colleen's time with Bill, and Wendy presented it to the director.

And then the other shoe dropped. Wendy explained the program the agency had laid out regarding Colleen's position as a rehab counsellor: five hours a day of direct work with Bill, one hour a day for planning, one hour a day for travelling, and a half hour of paid break.

"Why are there five hours a week allotted for planning?" I asked. "We already have a goddamned plan. I just want someone to follow it, stick to it, and make it work for Bill. Planning, my ass!"

I was only getting started.

"For this they allocate $59,000 per year? Oh yes, and the $3,120 for travel expenses, totalling more than $62,000 a year? They are going to use eighty percent of this funding, three times more than I'm earning right now, so I can go back to work full-time? And they will pay it to someone who has never done this job? They could have hired Jan, who knows Bill and his routine almost as well as I do for half that amount. It leaves very little money for new rehabilitation. Now I understand why we haven't got enough money for health care! This is insane, insane, insane."

No disagreement from Wendy.

COLLEEN'S FIRST TRAINING day in the first week of September was informative, at least for her. She hadn't realized what her day would involve.

"You'll need to help him to get up, go into the bathroom, and do his morning grooming," I said. "You might need to change the sheets; accidents do happen. He can't reach under the chair to do anything bottom wise, so you'll have to do that and apply skin cream wherever necessary."

She flinched at this revelation.

"Once you help him get dressed you'll need to use the lift to get him into his chair."

She looked shell-shocked.

My next surprise: Colleen had never used a mechanical lift. Good God! In unskilled hands, these things were dangerous.

Colleen offered some suggestions of her own.

I bristled, thinking, "Perhaps you might want to learn how he already does things before you presume you know better and start trying to make changes."

I wanted to cry — or scream, "What the hell have I gotten us into this time?"

We pressed on, working from *Bill's Home Care Book* to discuss the daily schedule, his daily food and drink list, and then the Ex N' Flex exercising machine and some of his physio exercises. I sensed she'd had no idea what this job would entail.

The first day finally ended. We hadn't come even close to covering a normal morning, but none of us had the stamina to continue. In two days she'd be back to learn more. Exhausted, I curled up with Bill and Jessie, looking for comfort.

AFTER GOING BACK and forth with several optional plans for how best to use Colleen's hours, Wendy and the agency's director brought the final decision to me: Colleen could work five hours a day for four days and stay until two o'clock in the afternoon. Now, instead of two people and a short nursing visit, Bill would have to endure at least three people and a nurse every day. Damn. When I pointed out that PSWs can't do transfers or pills in the morning or evening, I could see by her pinched mouth and furrowed brow that the director was getting fed up with my roadblocks.

"Bill needs the continuity of the daily morning tasks, the consistency of approach to meals, and the routine of his exercises and rest periods, or we'll both be sunk," I went on. "He can't deal with four or more people a day. Nor can I."

The director didn't seem to recognize how this plan impacted us. People who had never set foot in our home were making decisions about our lives based on policies, not needs. And between all the policy issues, I had to keep telling people not to call me "his primary caregiver." Especially in front of him. I was trying to be his wife.

Finally, bereft of any choice, I agreed to their plan.

35

ON THE ROAD AGAIN

It often seemed just as I hit rock bottom a trampoline magically formed beneath me. A few months earlier, at the end of July, I was feeling particularly low, still reeling from a long stretch of obstacles, and anxious about the promised funding. Then something amazing happened. The manager of the wheelchair transport company called. An elderly client had a used wheelchair-accessible van for sale. Six thousand dollars. Were we interested? Were we? Oh yes!

I hung up the phone, anxious, both positively and negatively. I could almost taste the freedom a van would give us. But I could also taste the bile welling up in my stomach as I contemplated the cost. I explained the situation to Bill because I wanted him to be part of the decision-making process, to feel he was taking part in running our life. We were exuberant as we talked about the various outings we could go on and the freedom we would have.

The owner brought the van over Saturday morning. I wheeled

Bill out to the driveway to see it. He looked it over like the car fiend he had always been. He couldn't kick the tires, but he did give them a good inspection. He eyed the condition of the body, looked over the paint, and watched as I opened the hatch at the rear. It was hydraulic, and he would be able to put it up and down with the remote button himself.

We had discussed the price. He thought it was fair. Now, after seeing the van, I couldn't be certain if he had actually been taking all this in and processing it normally, but together we agreed to make the purchase. It would be a huge gift that would keep on giving. Within thirty-six hours, the credit card was maxed out, again.

Getting Bill into the van was a little more taxing than I had anticipated. When we put the ramp down it seemed a relatively low incline. Pushing Bill up the ramp, I was shocked by how high it was. I had a split second in which I could foresee us careening backward down the ramp, him rolling over me and crashing into the garage door.

That was enough to get me the hell up the ramp. I got a wheel stuck on one of the metal tie-down straps. No choice but to back ever so slightly down the ramp and try again. This time I tripped, shoving the chair forward with considerable speed and force. I was getting frazzled, but Bill said, "woman driver," which me laugh, grateful again for his humour and his faithful support.

After much trial and error, the tie-downs and his seat belt were secured. I belted myself into the driver's seat. Brenda and Jessie came along for the ride. We were off.

First stop? The Tim Hortons drive-through for the first time in two and a half years. Yahoo! Canadian maple donuts, Bill's favourite, and drinks were acquired, and we set off to the countryside. We could go wherever we wanted and stay as long as we wanted. This was a gift from God. We talked about all the places we passed, the trees, the beautiful gardens, and the beautiful blue water of the bay.

I had to remind myself to stop looking in the rear-view mirror to check on Bill's position. After a lengthy cruise, during which I felt I'd gotten the hang of driving a van, it was time to return home. As I turned the last corner onto our street, Bill let out an exclamation. His chair has toppled sideways.

"Wheelie!" he said, with enough enthusiasm to let me know he was okay.

Note to self: Must learn to use tie-downs properly.

We were all terribly impressed by how well the maiden voyage had gone. I knew how greatly the van would expand Bill's world. Our world.

Many days we ventured out to new places as well as old places nearly forgotten. There were concerts in the local park on Sunday evenings in the summer and car shows at the farmers' market. We even went to the movies, a favourite activity of ours in the past. Bill was mesmerized by *March of the Penguins*. I was mesmerized by him.

Most outings were relatively smooth, and we got more adventurous. Kevin invited us to join him and his family at his campsite on the waterfront, and we took up the challenge. The provincial park was beautiful and had been one of our favourite hiking areas. Driving through the heavily treed road into the park, we saw a number of deer and stopped to watch two pairs of swans in the marsh. The deep greens and yellows of the foliage gave the park a mysterious and peaceful ambience. We drove the trail very slowly, savouring all the details we had missed for so long.

Kevin was delighted to see Bill in this "outward bound" environment. We pulled chairs up close to the water's edge and found ourselves enveloped in a circle of friendship, something we hadn't experienced for quite some time. It was glorious to watch Kevin and Bill involved in a conversation about the sunset over the lake. Their shadows were huge, spreading along the grassy edge of the shore, but not as huge as this experience. I captured it on film, another Kodak moment.

Brenda and Jessie came with us to see the Air Force Pipe and Drum Band. Brenda hauled folding chairs, snacks, and drinks out onto the sun-drenched lawn. Sitting in his chair, Jessie on his lap, Bill was not very different from anyone else in the audience. He tapped his toes and clapped his hands and even sang and hummed along to some favourite tunes.

At the end of that summer, the cadet camp held a special event: a sunset closing ceremony on the parade square. Having been a cadet instructor, Bill was very keen to attend, so off we went in the van.

It was breathtaking. Hundreds of young people paraded into the square. In the shadow of the white stucco military buildings, under the arch of the parade square, they demonstrated the multitude of drills and marches they had mastered in a summer of training, dedication, and camaraderie. The drills were interspersed with a dozen musical exhibitions, mainly by groups of young people who had never met before this camp started. Bill watched every step of every drill, nodding approvingly.

He commented on the number of women cadets. "About time," he said.

Bill was definitely pro-feminism.

It was 2005, the Year of the Veteran. Nearing the end of the ceremony, dozens of these fine young people went into the audience, putting a memorial ribbon and medallion over the heads of those they presumed to be former military and veterans. As a young woman laid a ribbon around Bill's neck, she saluted him. He sat straight as a rod, saluting her in return. Old habits die hard. Tears filled my eyes to see my husband display so beautifully who he had been, who he still was.

When I was moving up the ramp into the van, he said quietly, "Our future is in good hands."

SEPTEMBER WAS ONGOING training time with Colleen. I tried to be positive, but it was impossible to move forward while spending so much time demonstrating, over and over, things that were second nature to Jan and me. I was exhausted from explaining every minute detail and how each one played into our overall goals. Some days were reasonably good, but some were desperately discouraging. I tried to let go of the resentment I felt about doing this training. Jan would have just taken over, and I'd already be back to work. Dear God, why was this system so convoluted?

Judy and one of Bill's brothers, Hector, came to visit late that month. They brought fun and laughter of a different kind into our home.

Great meals were synonymous with Judy's visits. She brought an array of Bill's favourite seafood and preserves from the Maritimes. Each meal was a feast for him, things I never could have cooked. They relished watching him devour these treats.

One day Hector bought a scarecrow for the yard. He set it out in the grass where Bill could see it when he got up from his afternoon nap. The moment Bill saw it, he said, "Looks just like Sarah McCrae. She was the girl who cooked at the hotel when we were kids. She was always stirring the pot on the stove and scratching her arse at the same time."

We all went into hysterics, with Judy and Hector assuring me it was a true story.

We drove to a waterfront park for a "hike." Ice cream, always Bill's weakness, was the main goal, but we included a marvellous stroll along the water's edge. It was a beautiful pathway, stretching for miles. Jessie alternated between perching on Bill's knee as his guardian, and roaming the path with Judy. For a while, we all forgot how abnormal our normal life really was. We were just like anybody else, out enjoying a beautiful evening and good conversation.

Hector and Judy updated us on all the goings-on in their lives. We watched the ducks and geese diving for fish and laughed as Jessie tried to catch them. I videotaped much of the outing. Bill would be able to watch it again and again if he forgot they'd been to visit. After they left, he indeed did forget. Not at all unusual. The video worked its magic, though. Once we watched parts of their visit a few times, it was locked into his memory, at least for a while. It had been an incredible visit.

36

AT CROSS-PURPOSES

THE LATE AUTUMN OF 2005 brought another discovery. The fitness centre right at the end of our street had a pool and an antiquated but functional hydraulic lift. I checked it out thoroughly, and Frank agreed to try it with Bill. Because we could meet him there, using the van, the whole process became simpler, took less time, and was far less costly. It had been months since Bill had been in the water, and he had missed it a lot.

It was out of the question to have Frank come more than once a week. It would have been beyond our budget, and it required a half-hour drive each way for Frank, who was coming on his lunch hour as it was. It forced me to get into the water with Bill myself two other days of the week. We managed surprisingly well, and I soon developed an enthusiasm for the water, at least with Bill.

Getting Bill in and out of the van was a cinch compared with getting him in and out of the pool, though. The hydraulic lift was a metal post, about five feet high, anchored into the pool deck. It had an arm that swung out over the pool. I used our fabric sling, fitting it to go under him in the lift's chair. Once on the pool deck, Bill and I hooked the loops of the sling onto the arm of the lift and pumped the hydraulic lever to lift Bill out of the chair.

Once he was high enough, I swung him out over the water and prayed he wouldn't decide to reach forward. I jumped into the water, trying to keep him steady at the same time. We counted to three and then released the lever to lower Bill into the water.

The first few times I was overzealous. He landed quickly, splish splash, went under, and surfaced coughing, spitting, and laughing. Once I mastered a slower descent, I was able to unclip the sling, hold onto Bill while he floated off it, and then heave the sling onto the pool deck. Often, mid-flight, Bill would announce, "Here comes the stork." There was a notable resemblance. After just a few visits, Bill was waving and talking to the now familiar regulars.

Going twice weekly, we perfected some incredible maneuvers. If I put my arms around Bill's neck and my feet just above his knees for weight, he could walk back and forth across the pool, supporting me and himself. We also got to slip in some hugs on the way. His balance was coming back extremely well, although he continued to list a little to one side. We started using pool noodles and played our own version of water polo, pushing a medium-sized ball back and forth.

Being in the pool was productive and entertaining for both of us. Bill laughed and splashed me and made funny faces. We'd have been great six-year-olds together. I loved to have people come to watch, so Bill could show off. It was worth any amount of effort to have this much fun.

COLLEEN AND I were still very ill at ease with each other. I didn't see any great skills surfacing, and often I sensed we were not working toward the same goals. Mine was to get her so adept with Bill's program that I could return to work full-time and feel he was in good hands. Hers seemed to be to reinvent *Bill's Home Care Book*.

In mid-October I came to understand my disquiet. Colleen proudly showed me how she had taken all the information I'd assembled over two and a half years and reformatted it. There were very few changes, but every detail was broken down into even more minuscule steps. As I thumbed through her version, I realized it was even more intimidating than mine.

"Laid out this way it is a better training tool," she said, a little too arrogantly for my liking.

"Why do we need a better training tool?"

"For training the new staff Bill will have."

"What new staff and what training are you going on about?"

"Well, we'll be getting at least eight new people thoroughly oriented over the next six weeks. With my breakdown of each task, they will be able to follow everything step by step."

"What the hell are you talking about? Why would we want eight new people to go through training? And even if we did, why would it be done in such a short time? And no one could possibly memorize all the minutiae in there!"

I was jabbing my index finger at her training manual but really wanted to jab it into her eye. I wondered if this accounted for the hours of very expensive planning time.

"Once several people are up to speed, I will schedule them to work with Bill and me. Once they all are well versed, I will be the on-call person if they encounter any problems. They will be able to call me anytime. On my cell. That will take the pressure off you. You won't have to train any of these new people. Won't that be wonderful?"

It was crystal clear to me that we truly were at cross-purposes. Not only were we not on the same page, we weren't even in the same book!

After two months of essentially being trained by me, Colleen was telling me the goal was to train six or eight new staff. And she would be doing the training, she who still couldn't use a lift, wipe shit off a backside, or add any new skills to Bill's life. She would be unaware of any progress he was making, or what skills he was losing, except as reported by her underlings.

Carefully, and quietly, I explained *my* goals and *my* understanding of her position: to have one main person, herself, work with Bill, long term. Evidently that was not her understanding. I asked her to consider my next comment very seriously: "If you aren't planning to be here for the long haul, we have an enormous conflict."

I met with Wendy later that day and let her have it with both barrels.

"What are those freaking idiots in your agency thinking? They're supposed to be brain injury experts. Do they still not grasp the need for a very small number of people on this team? Did they not understand Dr. Carlson's recommendation that Bill have a one-on-one person for continuity? Do they not grasp the cost to Bill every time someone new starts? Do they not understand that this girl is not up to doing the training? She can barely do most of it herself. What are they thinking?"

Wendy suggested a meeting with the main players from the agency, the Ministry of Health, and the Community Care Access Centre might help. I told Colleen that by the meeting date I needed to know if she was prepared to stay on as the rehab counsellor. I did not want a trainer. I wanted a person who would work one-on-one with Bill and train new people only as needed. As I explained this to her, I recalled how many times I had tried to make this point during the last two and a half years.

I asked Wendy, "Why is my communication so poor? Why am I still begging for what is best for Bill? Why is there so much offered that we don't need but so little of what we do?"

Neither she nor I could answer the questions.

37

BUREAUCRATIC COMPOST

WENDY WAS ABLE TO organize a meeting at the RCBIS satellite office in Belleville. Besides her, this would include Dawn, the RCBIS director; Colleen; Dr. Carlson, the RCBIS neuropsychologist; our CCAC case manager and her supervisor; and, via conference call, a rep from the Ministry of Health and Terri from Chedoke, who had initiated this special funding.

I had put all my thoughts, questions, and concerns on paper to avoid getting sidetracked or losing my temper. I gathered up my "screw you" picture album and Bill's oil painting for show and tell.

After introductions all around, I launched into my agenda. I thanked everyone, acknowledging that they had started out trying to do something wonderful for us. I handed our pictures around the table. I wanted the managers to see Bill the person, not just a file. I propped his painting on a chair, almost daring anyone to think him unable to live a quality life.

"As you all know, Bill and I left Trenton Hospital nearly two and a half years ago. There was no hope or help there for him, and I doubt that he would be alive today had he remained there. Since then we have developed a very detailed, and pretty successful, amateur home rehab program. With the help of the Access Centre, and after a lengthy struggle with agencies, we now have two main people who are very skilled at working with both of us. Getting the service providers to understand the value of continuity in staff was a huge task. I think this would be important for anyone with complicated conditions, but for acquired brain injury it is essential. But you all know that. This is *your* expertise.

"I am extremely grateful for this funding. I believe that all of you want the same thing I want, which is that this money be used to provide the things we need to continue to improve life for Bill. That it be used to do what it was intended for: to help him, us."

I launched into my thoughts on the difficulties attached to his funding.

"Why is it labelled 'for respite'? The Ministry of Health's definition of respite refers to paying for the patient to go into a nursing care facility for a week or more to provide the 'caregiver' a rest. I know you will understand why that is not an option for me. Respite for *me* means competent help for him that would allow me to go back to work full-time. I know that some disabled people, deemed able to 'self-direct' this funding, are allowed to hire the people they choose. Parents are able to hire staff privately with this type of funding and get far greater value. I feel as though I, or any other spouse, am not trusted to do the best for him. But I can assure you that I would not be spending more than sixty thousand dollars a year for one worker."

I tried not to sound sarcastic, but likely was not successful.

"Every person with an acquired brain injury is unique, as is every relationship. So I hope you'll understand when I tell you the hardest thing I do in my life is leave Bill and go to work in Toronto, entrusting his care, safety, and well-being to others. The notion of this funding paying for Bill to be sent to a nursing home for a few weeks for me to have respite is entirely opposite to our needs. The respite I have sought has always been about physiotherapy, daily life skills, equipment, and anything else that would help us attain the highest quality of life possible. More time away from Bill is not my idea of respite.

"We've established a program and routine we know works. We get practical problem-solving help from Wendy. Linda has fought to provide good home care staff, and the fewest, for Bill. He has accomplished so much. Impressive gains for a man given no option but a nursing home just two and a half years ago. We've learned the hard way that adjusting to each new person brings an inevitable setback in Bill's progress. It takes ages for him to connect with someone new, and longer for them learn his routine. Rarely do I ever get to a comfort zone, with a few wonderful exceptions. With each new person we lose a lot of quality time.

"The major decisions about how to use this funding were made without our true needs being considered. We've been asked to fit our very square circumstance into a very round solution. Our real needs would have used only half of this funding. The mandate we're forced to accept uses all of it. It can't be used for vital rehab expenses like physiotherapy, art lessons, equipment, swimming, transportation, and a skilled worker. What we can have is many hours of what we don't need.

"My position was never about the money until I learned that sixty thousand dollars is allocated for a counsellor to work twenty hours a week with Bill, hands on. We don't need a planner. We don't need any more chiefs. We don't need any more people telling us what we need. This is not about Colleen, except in that she isn't qualified, other than on paper, to do this job. She earns three times as much as I do, and three times as much as Jan, and she can't do the job as well as either of us.

"I would have allocated twenty dollars an hour to have Jan for many more hours, topping up what we already receive from home care. We would spend this money on physiotherapy. It has already proven invaluable. We'd use it for transportation, and recreational programs, which are true respite for both of us. But these appropriations do not fit the mandate. What does seem to fit is a huge expense for little value. The Ministry of Health is paying thirty-two dollars an hour to an agency for a support worker who, in fact, makes twelve dollars an hour. They pay fifty-six dollars an hour to an agency for a practical nurse, which we don't need nearly as much, who makes twenty-four dollars an hour.

"If I was directing this funding, we would obtain far more value for the money spent, and some other poor soul with an acquired brain injury could have help, too. I am begging you to advocate for us to have this money better spent. I am begging you to advocate for changes to meet the specific needs of an individual case. I am begging you to help us use this money better for Bill. Please."

AFTER TWO HOURS and much lecturing about the rules, nothing changed. This money was for very specific uses, as defined by the Ministry of Health.

It could not be used for physiotherapy, as that could be provided by the Access Centre. (It didn't matter that there was no one there who could do what Bill needed or that it could only be a maximum of one hour a week.)

It could not be used to hire Jan, because the rehab counsellor job remained a union position (even though they had no one in-office with the appropriate skills for this circumstance).

It could not be used for equipment. The Assistive Devices Program provided mobility equipment. (But not a standing frame, or an Ex N' Flex, or transportation, or a mechanical lift, or an electric hospital bed that goes up and down.)

It could not be used for any of the expenses for travel to the pool, or painting, or anything recreational.

Another day away from Bill and nothing accomplished, nothing gained. Just another heap of bureaucratic compost. Take it or leave it.

Driving home I tried to see the other side. Was I really so demanding? Was our routine really so complex? I raged to myself about the bureaucracy of our health care system. We would have been so much better off and accomplished so much more if the upper echelon had simply listened better and used some discretionary judgment. My conviction that much more could be accomplished with taxpayer money held like concrete. I believed strongly it would have provided extra help to two individuals with unusual needs at home.

Although I was relieved when Colleen decided to resign, the timing was dreadful. I was just entering the busiest five weeks of the year at work, and suddenly we needed to fill in Colleen's block of time. My first call was to Jan to ask her how she could make this work. She said she would try to do some trades in her schedule. My next call was to Wendy. She knew about Colleen's resignation and was already problem solving. She would also juggle her appointments to make extra time with Bill.

38

ALL I NEEDED TO KNOW

LINDA, BILL'S HOME CARE case manager from CCAC, called to say she had a new PSW lined up.

"I'd like you to meet her. She has a very suitable background, but I'd like you to explain your program to her. She's keen, and we can get her scheduled in very quickly."

Marie came to visit us the next evening. I explained the whole regimen, deliberately making it sound even harder than it was. She visited with Bill and me for a while and then said, "I really admire what you two are doing. I would love to take part in this."

I had a good feeling about her, and Bill said she seemed pretty funny. In his life, funny was a valuable trait.

With a new schedule up and working, training Marie was split between Jan, Wendy, and me, and she was quickly entrenched. I was quite at ease leaving Bill in her care, knowing she could, and would, call Jan for advice. Wendy taught her the most effective ways to interact with Bill, and maybe even with me! A nurse was still doing visits for catheters the days I worked, and finally the agency was doing its best to send the same person most of the time. We were indeed making progress. Marie was enthusiastic, Jan was impressed with this new person, and Bill was impressed with her, too. Finally, we could move forward again.

FOR MY BIRTHDAY at the end of November, Brenda bought tickets for the three of us to attend the St. Michael's Choir School concert at a church in Trenton. It was a beautiful winter evening as we set out in the van. One of our friends was an usher, and he seated us right at the front by the altar, the best seats in the house. As the lights dimmed, dozens of angelic boys and young men paraded by us. We were mesmerized by the crystal-clear voices and the magnificent music. I noticed Bill tapping his toes to the cheerful carols, bowing his head during the more solemn hymns. We held hands and again were transported, at least in spirit, back to a time when this would not have been an unusual outing. This was a very happy birthday indeed.

IT WAS TIME to start Christmas preparations in our house. Although we no longer hosted the family dinner mid-December, we still did considerable entertaining under the circumstances. The tree and the music were the main event for us, even more so now that the tree sat in the corner of our bedroom/living room. Dressed in eight hundred clear lights, it was stunning. A beautiful angel, saved from our first Christmas together, always sat prominently at the top. Carols played as Bill carefully unwrapped each gold or burgundy ball for me to hang. Strands and strands of golden beads and burgundy bows also adorned our creation. In the soft light it was enchanting.

We spent hours and hours by the fireplace during the month, sitting together in the quiet, soaking up the beauty. Many times I'd say my silent prayer of thanks for yet another beautiful season together, in our own home, with our life and our love.

Brenda and Bill had a new project. They made bird feeders from terracotta flowerpots. They placed and glued snowman faces and hands, lavished simulated snow on them, and tied birdseed to their bases. They had a grand time doing them together. Bill felt they were purposeful and therefore worth doing. It was also another good excuse to listen to music and eat Christmas cookies.

Family came for dinners and visits, which helped make the holidays seem normal. My cousin and her son visited, and our neighbours Al and Georgia joined us for wine and treats. They even brought a present for Jessie. It was placed under the tree with much ceremony, to be left there until Christmas morning.

Our tradition of opening gifts after midnight mass had changed. I couldn't stay awake that late any more, the effort to get to church was out of the question, and now it took forever for Bill to open his gifts. He'd never been one to rip through them haphazardly, but now every package had to be inspected, shaken, squeezed, and listened to. I laughed at him, asking what he heard.

"I hear all kinds of secrets."

"Did you hear how much I love you?"

He pointed to the gift at hand. "Not from this one, but maybe the next one."

His eyes twinkled. Mine got teary.

Dinner on Christmas Day was at Joyce and Earl's home. What a special Christmas gift it was for us to have our own van so we could go when we wanted and stay until we were good and ready to go home. We could relax and I could savour a glass of wine early on, a rare opportunity since I was, or course, the designated driver. The best thing about being with these friends was that they didn't care whether Bill was talkative or not.

Later that evening when we settled in our bed, Bill did the sweetest thing. He wrapped me in his arms, kissed my forehead, and said, "Thank you." I didn't know what I was being thanked for, but he was happy and content, and I was happy and content. That was all I needed to know.

39

ONLY TIME WILL TELL

The year 2006 rolled in, reminding me how long we had been living this new and very different life together. A new year always brought a renewed sense of optimism: fresh start, clean slate, enthusiasm. Three years had passed since we entered our adventure. Since returning home in 2003, Bill's abilities and improvements, though including lots of ups and downs, had been remarkable. This year held the promise of being the best yet.

After the holiday break, Bill got back into his routines quickly and easily. Jan, now our official full-time rehab counsellor, mentored Marie, who had a natural talent for getting the best out of Bill. Finally, I would be able to ease back into full-time work. Jan was a godsend and provided encouragement for me, often without even knowing. I finally had faith in our support system.

Bill's days still varied: some exceptional, others not. Bill was happy when it went well, but never unhappy if it didn't. I envied his "disability," gift really, for living almost only in the present. My nemesis was any time Bill achieved less than the week before. Was another backslide lurking? Another infection just waiting to jump in? He had come so far, in spite of so many regressions, but I was always a little fearful a new problem would surface and cause another regression.

I LEARNED FROM Marie that another problem, a more sensitive one, had crept into our life.

"When you're away, your sister is too involved with Bill and me," she said. "She may mean well, but she sometimes interferes with our routine. I believe she's very worried about you, but she says you're too hard on Bill and try to control too much. I don't want to get in the middle here, so what should I do?"

She was indeed caught between a rock and a hard place: between two sisters and two very different points of view.

"That likely comes from listening to me rant about this system and sharing my stresses," I told Marie.

I had often worried that, when I talked about a new problem or miscommunication in the system, or other concerns, I would unwittingly leave myself open to others' opinions, criticisms, or judgments. But being second-guessed about Bill's well-being wounded me badly. My intuition regarding Bill was high. I trusted wholeheartedly that my decisions for him were as good as I could make. With the arguments and disappointments and setbacks I had gotten through, the last thing I needed to cope with was being undermined, especially by my sister. The notion that she might be seeking support for her own opinions and interfering with my decisions both hurt me and brought out the bitch in me.

Time to change the rules. I wrote new instructions in our book: "When I'm away, the curtain separating our area from the rest of the house is to be kept closed. At all times. No one is to pass through."

This put Jan and Marie in an awkward position, but it was my husband, my home, my rules.

As winter sailed fairly smoothly into spring, life got easier. There were no medical emergencies and things were calm, except for the tension between Brenda and me. The feeling that she and I were in a bizarre competition kept creeping into my mind.

Bill delighted in playing darts with Marie and improving his prowess with the punching bag. He'd sit for ages on the bed, and, with perfect balance, stretch way out to give it a left or right jab. Watching him follow three-step instructions was rewarding. But the look of achievement on his face: priceless. Many nights I would get a laughing report on his antics of the day.

Pool days continued to be our favourites. They were always fun, providing lots of laughter and great displays of progress. Walking back and forth in the pool with me perched on his knees, Bill's job was to look at the other side of the pool and get us there safely. My job was to be on guard for the first inkling he was going to dump us both. He had no sense of being in any way limited. What a godsend. Many of the regulars chatted with him, and he answered, or waved and smiled. He had his own fan club there.

Other aspects of our changed life still loomed like demons in the background. Living on so little sleep was taking its toll. There was always a stack of unpaid bills, and our home seemed to always be in disarray. I felt terribly isolated from friends, and reclaiming my career was proving to be more difficult than I had expected. I had become, in my eyes, a failure. I missed who I used to be, both at work and at home. I had always loved being Bill's wife and partner, and I wanted that life back. I didn't want to be this new me. But at the same time, I had not a single regret about our choice to come home. It was that schizofrantic person in my head who was messing me up.

One night Dr. Carlson called to see how we were making out, and how I was coping. I tried to be balanced in my comments, telling him about the new things Bill was doing, and how well the current team was working out, but there were also things that remained serious problems, despite the funding. Especially the financial aspects of therapy and equipment. I exploded when he said, "I understand your position, and I know it's an imperfect system."

"Well, goddamnit, you are the people who can change that!"

I was immediately contrite. He did not deserve my rudeness. He did understand my disappointment about the rules for the funding, and my opinion that so much of it was not being well used, and he was certainly still doing whatever he could to be supportive.

IN EARLY APRIL Bill got a dreadful cold. He hacked and coughed and wheezed and snorted. The protein shakes he drank every day increased mucous production, which made the coughing even worse. His coughing fits sometimes sounded more like choking. I was accustomed to this by now, but for Marie it was frightening. Mostly to put her mind at ease I asked Dr. Shirriff if he could come to check Bill. He agreed it was just a bad cold and told us what to look out for and to call in a few days if I was still concerned.

I hoped his opinion would relieve Marie's concerns, but unfortunately it did not. Just a couple of weeks later she told me she was leaving because of agency problems. I suspected it was more about the coughing and stress issues, but I couldn't change her mind. I was terribly disappointed because she had been a great asset to Bill.

Once again in need of a new PSW, I started interviewing. Any hint that the candidate wasn't receptive to a rehab environment, or had the wife-in-denial attitude, earned them a failing grade. It seemed harsh, even to me, but I was very short on time, energy, and patience.

The case manager arranged for two fellows to meet us, Jared and Phil. Both were polite and tried to communicate with Bill. However, I was wary of the agencies sending people who had no knowledge of rehab or brain issues, or who came expecting to do light duties or palliative care. Preconceived ideas and misinformation had been my nemesis for ages now.

While talking to Jared, I realized a gay man might be disturbing for Bill. This was an issue I had never thought about before. As Jared talked about his work background, it became apparent his experience was mainly in palliative care. Strike two. He seemed doubtful about the rehab information I was explaining. Strike three.

As I walked him through *Bill's Home Care Book*, explaining the intake/output sheet and the daily schedule of activities and exercises and defining clearly why it was so important it be adhered to, I saw a shift in his body language. Developing a rapport with Bill seemed a completely foreign idea to him. Strike four.

After he left, I asked Bill how he felt about this guy. He rolled his eyes to the ceiling and groaned, lifting his pinkie finger for emphasis. Decision made.

Phil, our second candidate, was a slight, short man in his late fifties or even early sixties, with a soft voice and rather nervous manner. As I went through our litany of background information, goals, philosophy, and schedules, Phil asked good questions and nodded appropriately. Knowing our choices were limited, I focused on the positives: He seemed open-minded, and although his background was not in rehab, he seemed genuinely willing and interested. All of us, Bill included, agreed to give it a try.

Phil came for a couple of training shifts with us, and while he seemed to grasp the concepts I heard that inner voice whispering, "Only time will tell."

But before he even got booked into the schedule, another problem reared its head.

40

AT MY OWN INQUISITION

IN MAY BILL STARTED having small seizures again. This time Dr. Spiller got him admitted to her hospital quickly and began the process of medication adjustments immediately. Thankfully, he was not nearly as unwell as he was during his other times there. This time he was in the neuro critical care unit for only a few days while staff did an MRI and conducted other simple tests.

Once the seizures were more controlled, Bill was moved to a private room. While the doctor waited for the results of the blood work and other tests, I waited anxiously for the MRI report. Regrowth of a tumour was always my principal fear. But the oncologist settled me down on that score.

"Well, Catherine, no notable change. There's still nothing to indicate any need for chemotherapy at this point."

Eventually a urinary tract infection was found to be the culprit, again.

The drive home that first Friday night was long and slow. I had made it a point not to call the hospital during my workday, trusting the staff would call if there was a problem. With Brenda and Jan each spending part of the day at the hospital with Bill, I'd been reasonably at peace through this particular day, but I was always anxious to get home and call for updates.

Dropping my bag and jacket on my way to the phone, I made my call to the nursing station.

"Nothing out of the ordinary today," said Bill's nurse.

Good. I asked about his blood work and some other incidentals, and thanked her. As I was about to end our chat, she said, "Tell your sister I put her letter to Dr. Spiller in the mail tube myself."

"Say that again?" I said.

She repeated herself.

"Why would you be sending a letter to Bill's doctor from my sister?"

The nurse began to stumble over her words, trying to explain her favour for Brenda.

"Why do I have the horrible feeling this can't be a good thing?" she said, and as she tried to apologize.

"It's not your fault," I said. "I'm sure you were just trying to help. No point in worrying anyway. It's already done."

What the hell had Brenda done? I stood immobile, still holding the phone. Fear and anger bubbled up like an oil strike. A kaleidoscope of her opinions, frequently differing from mine, flashed through my memory. All the small and large differences in how we saw Bill's home life. Although I believed my sister truly wanted the best for Bill, and probably for me, I was acutely aware of how different our perspectives were. I could only assume her letter was a criticism of what I was doing with Bill and included her opinions on how I should be doing it, otherwise it wouldn't have been a stealth project. Otherwise she would have talked to me before writing a letter to his doctor.

I tried to control myself to avoid storming through the door and beating the life out of her. I made my way upstairs to her bedroom door as I fought mightily to stay calm.

"The nurse wanted me to assure you she has forwarded your letter directly to Dr. Spiller," I said.

Shock, fear, and then "damage control" spread across her features.

"I didn't send a letter to Dr. Spiller."

"Well, the nurse said *my sister* did, and since you and Jan were the only people there today, I'm damned sure it wasn't her. I can't believe you would go behind my back like this to present your views to Bill's doctor. It isn't your place."

Retreating to the main floor, I tried to digest this new addition to my worry list. What devil had Brenda set in motion? Our altercations and differing opinions during the last two years washed over me. This was the ultimate betrayal.

THE ANSWER TO my question came on Monday morning when Dr. Spiller appeared in Bill's room. Her body language asked, "What is really going on in this man's life?" Her very direct gaze met my eyes, never flinching.

"I understand you've had mail," I said. "I don't even want to know what's in that letter, but please remember that it is one person's very different point of view."

The doctor immediately turned her attention to Bill.

"Hi, Bill, how are you doing this morning?"

"Not bad. I'm okay."

Then the questions for me began.

"Does Bill have a pretty strict regimen at home? Do you adjust his medications on your own? How are his spirits? Is he depressed, or sad? How much food and drink is in his diet? Does he have ulcers on his body?"

I answered the first questions in an even tone, but this last one pushed me over the edge. I knew where I stood now, and what the letter had implied. Suddenly I had to prove Bill wasn't being mistreated. I grabbed the sheets on the bed, yanked them off, and cast them onto the floor, exposing Bill's completely naked body.

"Does this look like someone who is being mistreated?" I asked.

I was immediately horrified that I had done something so insensitive to him, but I was at my own inquisition. Once someone, anyone, claims that a patient is being mistreated in any way, medical personnel must follow a protocol. Everything must be investigated, including the emotional and physical aspects of a patient. I valued this about the system, but having my commitment to Bill's life questioned, even for a minute, was soul-wrenching.

By the next day Dr. Spiller was in her usual open and forthcoming manner with me. I was relieved. I would not want her on the other side.

She speculated that perhaps Bill had SIADH (syndrome of inappropriate anti-diuretic hormone, a condition in which there is too much anti-diuretic hormone for a person's level of hydration). This was normally treated with fluid restriction, and that was the course she would follow. I was concerned because Bill's response to fluid restriction in the past had always been a severe drop in consciousness. This was partly why I was such a tyrant about his fluid intake at home. However, discussion was not going to change the plan.

Desperate for a second opinion, I called Dr. Shirriff. He knew I was afraid Bill would go into the deep zone again and advised me to speak to Dr. Spiller alone, not in front of a group of residents, and explain *why* I was so concerned.

When the opportunity arose I tried to be concise and clear. She still felt she was right, and so I relented. After all, I wasn't the doctor, and I did trust her. The next morning, though, as the neurologist rolled past, she casually remarked, "Change of plan. I've lifted the fluid restriction."

I never got a chance to ask why, but I wondered if she had discussed it with our family doctor. Within a few days, Bill was back up to par and discharged. Grateful, relieved, and anxious to get home together again, we kept our goodbyes short.

I still didn't know how to deal with the issues between my

sister and me. I was torn between my anger and frustration and feelings of betrayal and the many positive ways in which she actually did help Bill and me. In the end, by the time we settled into bed that night, I had realized it was better for Bill to have her here than not. I would try to learn to let sleeping dogs lie.

41

"I FEEL LIKE CRAP"

A HOSPITAL STAY ALWAYS created some regression for Bill, but this time there was much less than in the past. But because Bill was still a little fatigued, Jan and I agreed on a few minor changes in his daily routine, including using the mechanical lift for at least a few days. She would reiterate all of this when Phil arrived for his first "alone" shift, emphasizing the safety reasons for not doing pivot transfers.

I headed home from the city hopeful that these two very different men had had a comfortable time together. I shot into alarm as I entered the house. I knew something was way out of whack. Phil's demeanour increased my alarm. His hands were shaking, and he was almost chalk-white.

I spent my first few minutes with Bill, as usual.

"How was your day? Did you play with Jessie? Was she good today? Did it rain here?"

Bill answered, but seemed a little dazed.

Finally, pulling Phil into the front hall, I asked, "What is wrong?"

After a lengthy pause, he said, "Well, our afternoon went very well. Bill got through all his drinks, he finished his dinner without a huge amount of help, and we watched *Jeopardy* together. Things had been going so well I thought we could do a pivot transfer from the bed back to his chair. But once he was up, I guess our shoes must have gotten tangled. We both fell. But I really do think he is okay."

I wanted to slap him. Hard.

"Please show me exactly what happened," I said, trying not to sound angry or frightened, although I was both.

Phil demonstrated. My point about following instructions (and not second-guessing me) had fallen on yet another person who hadn't taken me seriously. The re-enactment showed exactly how their feet would have become entwined and exactly how they would have fallen over. Bill, nearly six feet three, was a foot taller than Phil. We could do these transfers because we'd been doing them for three years. We had a rhythm and routine. Bill was never uncomfortable being so close to me, but even with Jan and Wendy, both tall women whom Bill trusted, there was still a slight reluctance on his part to be in this almost intimate position.

I wanted to say, "Goddamnit! Why can't people just do what I ask them?" but kept the thought to myself, mostly for Bill's sake.

Bill's forehead was growing a goose egg. Landing face first on a concrete floor covered only with thin carpet was serious. He told me his back was stiff and a little sore. I wondered what else I should be checking for.

Phil went on his way, finally, and I poured myself a generous snifter of Grand Marnier and curled up with Bill and Jessie.

"Rough day, Hon?" the man with the egg-sized bump on his head asked. A master of understatement.

I e-mailed Phil the next morning to say he should make an incident report, and then called the case manager with what information I had. She sent a nurse to check Bill — and to teach me how to tell when Bill had a concussion and what danger signs to watch for.

Over the weekend we both needed to rest and relax and get over the physical and psychological events of Friday night. Frustration and anger mingled with worry. Each time I envisioned Bill's fall, my stomach lurched. How shocking it must have been for him. How many more problems would he suffer because of others' carelessness or poor judgment?

I drifted in and out of a daydream about how different Bill's circumstances could have been. Every ounce of my being still believed that if he'd been admitted to a rehabilitation centre for a few months, or even a few weeks, instead of the warehouse, he would have been dramatically farther ahead when he came home. I could have learned a lot from professionals who understood brain rehab. So many problems would have been avoided. I would have learned how to get appropriate people to work with him. The health care system would have saved money. Bill would have been spared so much. But all of this was moot now.

Bill recovered from the fall in a few days. I did not.

The case manager came to see us again. I knew she was running out of options, but I refused to have Phil back in our home again, and I hadn't heard from his agency about the fall.

"Do the home care agencies understand the impact of someone totally ignoring my information? How dangerous it can be?" I asked Linda. "Do they know how important trust is? I need and want to trust the people they send, but I rarely can."

When I calmed down she was able to tell me she had contacted a new agency, called Pathways, which frequently provided support to residents with brain-related problems in group homes. In three years I'd never heard of them.

"The staff have to be skilled in cognitive and physio work," she added. "They were not a possible source before because they were not awarded the home care contract by the Ministry of Health."

I was dismayed to realize that more competent and suitable help had been out there all along.

Jan worked overtime, physically and emotionally, educating

and training the new home support people from Pathways. We both found it much easier to work with people who already had experience with brain issues. Bill gradually regained most of the stamina and enthusiasm he had lost in the fall with Phil, but now he was even more reticent to trust strangers with transfers. I was, too, but June and July moved along with fewer ups and downs. And, with Jan established as the chief, I started to work full-time. Again.

Bill's regular Tuesday visits with Kevin continued, and summer provided more outdoor activities. Lawn darts, basketball, and "making Kevin chase" were still Bill's favourites. Trips around the neighbourhood to admire the gardens and enjoy the summer air were often part of their evenings. Those few hours every week, just hanging out with a friend, were special, and we both looked forward to them and valued Kevin's gift of himself.

In late June, David and Bill started another painting. "I'm going to paint the ocean and a lighthouse, Hon. Remember the one at the ferry? That's what I want to paint."

The reference to this landmark from his hometown told me exactly what the painting would look like. During most of their classes they talked, and painted, and joked, and repainted, although occasionally Bill would still withdraw. Normal life was returning, and The Ingonish Ferry Lighthouse was emerging.

By the first week of July, just as the new support helpers were settling in well, I got a phone call at work from Jan. I sensed immediately there was a problem.

"Catherine, Bill had a fall from his chair. It was an accident, I swear. I don't even know how it happened, it was so fast. He's got a cut on his head, but I cleaned it and I don't think it's bad. What do you want me to do?"

Her voice was quivering, squeaking. I heard the tears just below the words.

"Do you think he needs to go to the hospital? How does he seem to you, Jan?"

"I think he's okay. He doesn't seem disoriented or in real pain, but he is pretty shaken up. It's almost time for his rest. Maybe the PSW can let him sleep later than usual today?"

"Okay, Jan. You need to calm down. I know you are never careless or incompetent with Bill. Accidents are just that, accidents. Get him settled in bed, but ask the PSW to keep him awake. He can watch TV until I get home. Go home, have a drink, try to put this behind you, and start fresh tomorrow. I'll see you in the morning."

Once I got home, however, I was shocked when I saw the gash on Bill's head. It spanned five inches across the top of his skull. Dried blood was matted in his hair. May stomach heaved as I started to clip away a few hairs at a time to get a better look.

I couldn't figure out how he could get a cut like this right on the *top* of his head. It was in such a straight line. It just didn't make sense.

I tried to mask my feelings when I asked Bill how he felt.

"My head hurts. My back hurts. I'm really tired. Where's the puppy?"

They were all logical answers, so maybe there was no concussion. My questions mounted, though, as I wondered if I should I put him through a trip to the hospital. In the end I decided to watch him overnight and call the doctor in the morning.

Throughout the night I shifted Bill into different positions, watching for any signs of pain. There were quite a few, but his breathing and temperature remained normal. I took solace in that, but prayed, "Please God, let this be okay."

I studied the large bloodstain on the carpet. It was right beside the track for the patio door, even overflowing onto it. Bill must have been sitting near the door, reached to open it, and fallen on top of the track, headfirst. Nothing else could explain the point of impact or the blood pool. I knew how quickly it could happen. It had nearly happened to me many times. Poor Bill. Poor Jan.

First thing in the morning I called Dr. Shirriff. As I described the accident, he said he'd come to see Bill during his lunch hour. Although Jan's description of the accident didn't quite match what

I saw, I knew she wasn't lying. More likely she was terribly traumatized by what had occurred, and I wasn't going to berate her for a genuine accident. She was probably in worse shape than Bill. Her cut went much, much deeper.

The doctor's visit was both comforting and worrying. He checked Bill's eyes with a flashlight. No sign of concussion. He poked and prodded.

"Does this hurt, Bill? Does that hurt? Can you read the clock? Do you have a headache? Can you hear me clearly?"

Bill's answers were all affirmatives. Then he said, "I feel like crap. Does that count?"

He chuckled. Dr. Mike chuckled. I didn't.

"Well, Catherine, no signs of broken bones. No signs of serious damage. But try to keep him drinking. I don't want him to dehydrate. I'll get the lab to come and do a daily blood workup to make sure nothing else is going out of whack. Give him some Tylenol to reduce the pain, and I'll call you tonight. We just have to wait and see."

Over the second and third weeks of July, he sent Bill for x-rays of his back and chest to make sure pneumonia hadn't set in. A spinal compression showed up, but there was no way of knowing if it was from this most recent fall. Nothing serious was evident, except that Bill was recovering very slowly. My fears never abated. What if, what if, what if was a constant refrain.

One more conversation with Dr. Shirriff, and then one he had with Dr. Spiller, culminated in the decision that I would drive Bill to Kingston Hospital myself, present him at the ER, and get a CT scan done. Maybe it was more for my benefit than Bill's.

Off we went. Even allowing for the loading/off-loading process, the two-and-a-half-hour round trip, and the hospital processing, we were there and back in five hours.

The next day the oncologist called.

"Catherine, I just received a report on a CT scan done on Bill. I didn't have him scheduled. Why was it done?"

I told her what had led to the test.

"Well, there is a *speck* on Bill's CT. But the radiologist wouldn't have known a fall was the reason it was done. It's probably a tiny blood pool from the fall, but there is always the remote chance it could be the beginning of new growth. No way to tell for certain, but I'm going to schedule another scan for September 4. Keep me posted on any changes."

FOR THE NEXT few weeks, Bill progressed very slowly back toward normal. We followed our usual daily routines, but with great moderation. Inactivity had always increased weakness and fatigue, but we absolutely had to go slowly this time. Dr. Shirriff called or visited every other day. Bill's cut had healed quickly, but the rest of him was taking longer.

Small seizures started up again, barely discernible, but there. He was showing signs of dehydration again, and the lethargy that went with it. Dr. Shirriff prescribed an IV fluid line, saying, "The home care nurse will put one in and start a drip."

When the visiting nurse couldn't do it, Dr. Shirriff told us to take Bill to the ER at Trenton Hospital and have them put one in. He would order ambulance transport.

No problem. Jan would go with him and stay with him throughout the process. It shouldn't take long.

For once, things would be simple.

42

"MIGHT NOT BE GOING HOME"

On Friday, August 11, before starting my workday, I called the neurologist. The second Dr. Spiller answered her phone I launched into my reason for calling.

"Bill's having low-grade seizures again. Do you think we could increase the drug?"

She asked a few questions and then paused before saying, "I think it may be an absorption problem. I'd like to try a nasal gastric tube for a few days to check. If the seizures stop, then we know it's an absorption problem. If not, then an increase is the answer."

"He's at Trenton Hospital having an IV line put in today. Should we come to Kingston General to have the nasal gastric tube done?"

"That's not necessary. They can do it in Trenton since Bill's already there."

"I'd feel better bringing him to Kingston General."

"Catherine," Dr. Spiller said, "a first-year med student can do these. Ask the ER doctor to call me."

I could picture her exasperated but understanding expression.

I thought, but did not say, "Yes, but he won't have the benefit of a first-year med student here."

There are times when you have to trust, and this was just one of many. She said she would call Trenton hospital and make the arrangements for the NG tube insertion.

Seven hours later, Jan called to tell me that, because of the number of emergencies at the hospital, and Bill didn't qualify as one of them, they were still waiting, but she had to leave. The agency was sending a substitute to relieve her. I rescheduled my late appointments and left work quickly. A stranger sitting with Bill in the ER was better than no one, but not much better. When I arrived, the tube had just, finally, been inserted, and an ambulance was waiting to take us home.

It hit the fan just as the paramedics left our driveway. Bill was making a strange noise.

"What the hell does he have in his mouth?" I said.

I leaned in close to check and realized *it was the tube*. The end of the nasal gastric tube that should have been in his stomach was coming out of his mouth. In a panic I called the hospital and explained what I was seeing. The nurse on the phone sounded like she was making light of my concerns. I reminded myself she was accustomed to these things. But I wasn't. I was frightened, worried, and angry watching Bill enduring yet another assault.

"Just come back and we'll redo it," she said, as if going back to the hospital was a simple effort.

Another ambulance trip. Another lengthy wait, another upheaval. After three and a half years we were on a first-name basis with all the paramedics, and thankfully, without exception, they'd been wonderful. Always efficient, concerned, calming, and patient.

When we arrived, a different doctor was on duty. He knew little about the earlier circumstances. Explaining why we were back, and asking if anyone had x-rayed for tube placement after the first insertion, I immediately regretted my sharp tone of voice. I saw it did not sit well with him. Relinquishing Bill into his hands, I stepped from the room.

As a nurse went in, I said, "Bill's blood work, done by the lab at home this morning, showed his INR is very high today."

A high INR (International Normalized Reading) indicates a patient is in danger of a major bleed.

She bristled. A very short time (too short, judging by previous experiences) later, the doctor emerged, walked past me without comment, and disappeared. As I entered Bill's cubicle, my heart skipped. Bright red blood filled the tube.

"Oh my God, what happened?" I asked the nurse.

"Oh, don't worry, dear. Sometimes we get a small abrasion that bleeds."

"So you are assuring me this won't become a major internal bleed?"

My voice was more of a shriek. I was more frightened than I had been in a very long time.

"Don't worry, dear. It will be fine."

I wasn't convinced it would be fine, but no one else seemed concerned, and once again I reminded myself: You have to trust somebody.

It was midnight before an ambulance was available to take us home. Again. Bill had been in the hospital for most of the last sixteen hours. Carefully resettled at home by the paramedics, he was beyond exhaustion. I was relieved when he drifted off to sleep immediately. I imagined how the confusion and physical invasion of this day had affected him. I hoped he would sleep long and deeply, less aware of the intrusive procedures and the blood in this tube.

Curled around him on the bed, hugging him as close as possible, I wanted him to have some relief. And me.

I watched all night. The tube was still bright red, and I pictured Bill's body filling up with this blood that had no escape route. The tube was not open ended. It was capped when not being used to inject medication. With a high INR, blood does not coagulate and people can very quickly bleed out. Bill may well have bled out if the tube had not been capped, but instead he was bleeding internally. Late into the night I crucified myself with questions. Why in God's name had I let them send Bill home? Everything about this felt wrong. I knew enough, by now, to know what to be afraid of.

Saturday afternoon the IV pump stopped working. I couldn't restart it. I called the nursing agency. A supervisor was on call. She tried to instruct me over the phone: Push this button, push that button, turn this, wind that. To no avail. I wasn't getting the job done, and I was getting more upset and frantic by the minute. I had to beg her to come out to help me. Finally she agreed.

I watched her walk up the driveway with what looked to me like an arrogant and angry swagger. I tried not to react to that. Bill needed this woman's help, and so did I. After her fifth attempt to do what she had insisted over the phone was so simple, she checked the manual. No solution. She pushed buttons randomly as she quietly fussed and fumed. Finally she resorted to calling a technician, which took several calls and much waiting.

When the call came, she detailed her needs and gave this unknown technician Bill's name, address, and other private information. I heard her say to the anonymous technician, "Yes, he's a palliative."

I was devastated, and furious. Did she think Bill was deaf? Her callousness was unconscionable. As soon as she got the pump restarted, I ushered her out, hoping we would never see her face again. I didn't give a damn what kind of day she'd had, nor what else was happening in her job or her life. Her behaviour was cruel and insensitive. This was a supervisor? Dear God!

All Saturday night I watched the blood in the nasal gastric tube. By morning I realized this problem was not going to correct itself. I phoned the hospital and left a message at the inpatient nursing station for Dr. Shirriff.

"Please, please page him and give him my message," I said. "Tell him I called, that Bill is in trouble, and this is an emergency."

The nurse said, "If it is an emergency you need to come to the ER."

"No, thank you. We have this emergency because of your hospital." The only person in that building I trusted now was Dr. Shirriff.

Within the hour the weekend on-call doctor phoned. When I explained what was happening, she told me Dr. Shirriff was out of town for the weekend but she would try to reach him for advice. Within minutes the phone rang again.

"Catherine, it's Mike Shirriff. What the hell happened?"

I gave him all the information I could. He was away at a hockey tournament and wouldn't be back until late Sunday night. He asked me a few questions, including what was coming out of the tube.

"I'll call and arrange for a reverse suction machine. They'll get it to you and set it up as soon as possible."

Would it suck out the blood that was pooling inside Bill's body? I didn't ask.

He called back at midnight to confirm that the machine had been delivered and set up, and to get an update.

"Why didn't the ER doctor just start the reversing process?" I asked him. "Why didn't he put Bill on frozen plasma right away? Why didn't he take responsibility for this screwup? He could have started to fix this immediately. Instead, he sent Bill home. To do what? Bleed to death?"

This time I was not yelling. Not even angry. I was beyond those emotions.

"I don't know, Catherine. But I'm truly sorry."

At five on Monday morning, August 15, Dr. Shirriff called again. He asked me to describe what was in the tube. Did the stuff look black, like coffee grounds? It certainly did.

"Get him to the hospital. I'll be in later."

Before being admitted to Dr. Shirriff's care, Bill was examined in the ER. Again. The nurse tested for MRSA because he had been in another hospital within the previous three months.

I chuckled, in my newly cynical way, and said, "If he has it we might all be in big trouble. Dozens of hospital and home care people have dealt with Bill since then."

I really wasn't expecting it to be a positive test, and neither was she. Bill was not isolated; no one donned the gowns and gloves.

The reverse suction process had been working. But the fluid coming out had changed from black to green. The colour of infection. Dr. Shirriff explained that Bill's blood tests did indeed show some kind of infection. He prescribed a stronger antibiotic.

Late that night I talked to Bill, whose eyes were closed.

"Once they get this mess cleared up we can head home, Hon. Only a few days, hopefully."

A nurse, overhearing this, leaned across the bed and said. "You know, dear, he might not be going home."

I winced. Was she a fortune-teller? Did she think her comment helped Bill or me? Didn't she know it is better to be hopeful than not?

By Wednesday the suctioning was discontinued, and Bill's regular medication and liquid food were restarted. The doctor, addressing my concern about Bill's not getting enough nutrition, asked for the dietitian's input. She agreed and carefully increased the quantity of food.

43

THE LAND OF DENIAL

"I FEEL LIKE CRAP," Bill told me as he woke on Thursday morning. A sure sign he was coming around again. Before most people were even out of bed, Dr. Shirriff arrived on his morning rounds. His news was that the infection seemed to be turning around, and if things continued on the upswing, Bill could likely go home Friday afternoon. I breathed a huge sigh, of relief, gratitude, and exhaustion.

As I left to go to work, Jan arrived to replace me. I was always concerned Bill would wake and not remember where he was, and why.

That day, that night, and Friday morning, things were still on track. Dr. Shirriff came in again and said he'd leave the prescriptions and any other information for me to pick up when I came to get Bill after work. Anxious to put this all behind but confident we were going to win another battle, I left for work.

Dr. Shirriff called me at three o'clock.

"Catherine, Bill's white blood count has gone up again, and we still haven't found the specific infection. I think he should stay here until we're absolutely certain it's totally under control."

His tone was very serious.

Trusting his advice, I said, "It's your show."

Over the weekend of August 20–21, he determined that Bill had developed pneumonia and had tested positive for MRSA. There were antibiotics for pneumonia but little choice of effective treatment for MRSA.

"Shit," I thought.

Now, on Monday, the staff donned gowns and gloves and masks. I found it amusing in a black sort of way. These same people had been taking care of Bill and other patients for days, unprotected. Now that there was proof, all precautions must be taken. Too little too late. I wondered why the test for this nasty bug, an inexpensive and noninvasive swabbing, wasn't done as a matter of routine when anyone *leaves* a hospital. They had it backwards, as far as I was concerned.

Dr. Shirriff was doing a juggling act, trying to balance the antiseizure medications with a number of antibiotics, nutrition, and God knows what else. By midweek things looked significantly worse. Every few hours the details changed from slightly better to slightly worse, then back to slightly better. I struggled to be hopeful. Really struggled.

On Wednesday afternoon, the doctor came to Bill's room. From his grim expression I knew I didn't want to talk to him here, even though Bill was asleep. We moved to the "quiet room" reserved for people who are grieving. It was appropriate. I was grieving.

"This infection is not turning around, and I'm running out of ideas," he said. Staring into my eyes, he said, in a quieter voice, "You seem like you are reaching the end of your rope."

My answer was out of my mouth before it even registered in my brain.

"I am at the end of being able to watch Bill struggle any more. I don't think he can win this one."

I could feel the tears sliding down my cheeks, and my eyes ached. Fireworks exploded in my head. Was that me speaking? But I knew, in my soul, that it was exactly what I thought and felt. I knew there wasn't much working in our favour now.

The doctor, who had seemed such an adversary just three short years ago, walked me gently through the possible scenarios, talking openly and with great compassion about what might come next. He would continue to try to fight for Bill, but he wasn't hopeful.

My final request of him was, "I don't want you to stop trying one second too soon, but I don't want you to keep trying one second too long. I am sorry to put this responsibility on you, but it is now your call."

Wednesday night I knew it was time to be direct with Judy. I tried to be honest about Bill's condition, but neither optimistic nor pessimistic. There was always a chance of improvement, but not a great one. She would call the family. Thursday morning she called. She would be flying in early Saturday morning. I was grateful, and hopeful. With her here, things might get better.

Thursday brought a very slight improvement in Bill, at least to my eyes. I called my cousin Sue from the hospital, as I did most nights. She would call our family. After we talked, and cried, and talked some more, she said, "I will still be praying for Bill tonight, Cath."

"This time let's pray for what is really best for Bill, whatever that is." I was surprised to hear myself say this. I was, of course, praying that God would think recovery was best.

The night was uneventful. I slept in short segments, resting my head in the cradle of his arms, needing to be held. The night nurses came in and out as they needed, but mostly we were alone in a darkened, quiet womb.

The doctor's morning visit revealed nothing new. Nothing worse, which was good. I was sufficiently optimistic, when Jan arrived, that I decided it was okay for me to go to work. I left the hospital around six o'clock in the morning. The drive to work went unnoticed. My mind was always on the next step, the next question, the next issue.

But had I finally reached the Land of Denial?

44

A BEAUTIFUL LIFE TOGETHER

As I opened the door at work on Friday morning, the phone was ringing. I'd grown to hate that ring, always fearful it was the harbinger of bad news. The unit clerk from the hospital said, "Dr. Shirriff doesn't think Mr. MacLeod is doing very well."

"I'm on my way."

When I arrived back in Bill's room, he didn't seem any different from when had I left earlier. What was I not seeing? Of course, I didn't know what the blood work or other information showed. What I did know was that, if Dr. Shirriff, after coming to check on Bill again, asked the unit clerk to call, then this is where I was meant to be.

Outside the sky was bright blue full of billowing white clouds. A brilliant sun had risen directly over the golf course I could see from Bill's window. Inside was a bleak picture of grey and black and sadness.

I put my head down, resting it in the cradle of his arm, trying to capture this feeling of physical closeness, to commit it to memory. All I wanted to do was crawl in and hold on. I did. I felt Bill shift to accommodate me.

For so long it had been about us being together, fighting on, battling the real and imagined foes, "till death do us part." I realized, in excruciating pain, this would be the hardest goodbye of my life. I knew Bill had nothing left to fight this. Whatever the unseen enemies in his body were, they were going to win, this very day.

Reliving the memories of our life, I shared them with Bill:

"Hon, you have been the most treasured gift in my life. You were so big and strong and protective of me. Sometimes in these last years I lost that picture completely, as if our whole life was only this most recent chapter. But it was only a small part of our time together. Remember when we looked through all our albums last week? We lived a beautiful life together, didn't we? I never imagined it would be ending like this, though.

"I always respected and admired you, but even more now because of how you lived these last few years. You put your heart and soul into it, didn't you? How did you manage not to be angry all the time? I always tried to imagine what it was like for you to be trapped in this situation. How could you still be funny? And not hate me all the times I got impatient with you? If I got frustrated when you couldn't do something, you always forgave me. I hope my stresses didn't hurt you. For all the arguments I had so many times, with so many people, it doesn't matter now whether I was right or wrong. And I was both.

"Now I understand that saying, 'If only I knew then what I know now.' I will always regret I didn't know information that could have saved you from so much. I would have fought a lot harder a lot earlier. Maybe I wouldn't have had to waste so much time and energy finding our way through the maze. I just didn't know.

"Thank you for a love and a life well spent."

45

THE UNDERLYING CAUSE?

ON FRIDAY, AUGUST 25, 2006, my husband, life partner, and confidant died in our local hospital, the result of a simple, but botched, hospital procedure.

I wish I could end this book on a more hopeful, loving note, but that would be a disservice — to Bill, to me, to anyone reading this book — for the story of the last years of my life with Bill is meant to be a cautionary tale, a warning that our health care system has some deep flaws, that it is not always as truthful and open as we would like to believe.

Which was underscored for me by one of the standard post-mortem forms, which read:

Cause of Death: pneumonia.
Underlying Cause of Death: brain cancer, 1992.

"Are you kidding me?" I said to Dr. Shirriff. "Bill was released from follow-up testing in 1997, five years after his first operation. And for ten years there had *never* been any evidence of cancer after the surgery and radiation."

From my point of view, even the surgery that started *this* story, ten years later, in 2002, wasn't the underlying cause of death.

"Well, Catherine, the premise is that if Bill hadn't had that brain tumour in 1992, he would likely not have been rendered susceptible to another one, or the problems that went with it."

Like a nasty little terrier, I barked, "Do you honestly believe that if the ER doctor had acted effectively as soon as he saw the bleed he caused by the tube he had just inserted down Bill's throat, and had started the process to stop the bleeding — instead of sending us home with an enormous problem — that Bill would have been lying in a bed in this hospital two weeks later dying of pneumonia?"

The doctor did not raise any protest or argument. He merely said, with intense honesty, "I am truly sorry."

FROM MY PERSPECTIVE, the underlying causes of my husband's death were several: that simple, but botched, procedure, horrendous miscommunication all around, and the many, many things I didn't know about the workings of health care.

For weeks I struggled with the fear that the ER doctor who caused the bleed would not be held to account for his neglect. I sent a letter to the hospital's Chief of Staff, asking him to investigate. My first letter was ignored. My second letter was ignored. My third letter went by registered mail. What I desperately wanted was an apology. An assurance that this wouldn't happen to someone else.

The response I got, finally, was, in short, "There is no indication in the records that this incident happened." (I didn't know the administration would never apologize, if only out of fear of litigation.) But the response led me to a search of Bill's medical records, from both hospitals. You have to pay for copies of everything you want, and it's not inexpensive, but for me it was worth it.

In October 2006, as I searched through the mountains of paperwork, the pieces of our puzzle began to fall into pace. I would see the neurosurgeon's report from February 20, 2003, to the ER doctor in Trenton, which said that Bill likely had experienced a grand mal seizure before waking up that morning. It also noted that the seizure could have been related to SIADH (syndrome of inappropriate diuretic hormone secretion) as well as to an adverse reaction to Decadron, the anti-swelling steroid medication Bill was being given. This last item was an issue I raised a number of times over the months of February and March, only to be repeatedly brushed off by residents and nurses alike.

Unfortunately, I didn't have a copy of that report in February 2003. Apparently the doctors at Trenton Memorial either didn't read it, or chose to ignore it.

And I didn't know — again until I was able to read the medical records — that the resident, whose first language was not English, when writing Bill's Discharge papers from KGH had mistranslated the oncologist's statement: Rather than indicating that Mr. MacLeod had no signs of tumour left to treat, and hence that chemotherapy was not called for at this time, she wrote: "Patient is not a candidate for chemotherapy." That single sentence said, to everyone who read it, "Patient is terminally ill."

I had always wondered why the neurology team, back in 2003, had been so quick (four weeks!) to label Bill as "unlikely to benefit from rehabilitation," and why Bill's most important doctors, the neurosurgeon and oncologist, had not been included in that all-important meeting — the family meeting — to decide Bill's future. Our future. To this day I often wonder if their opinions on prognosis and management had even been sought.

It was only much later that I learned of the urgency placed on all hospitals by the Ministry of Health to get patients off "acute care" hospitals' budgets as fast as possible. Money before care?

IN THOSE RECORDS I also read, in the physiotherapist's report, from that first week in Complex Continuing Care in Trenton: "Wife is unrealistic." Rather than find out for herself, or try to help us, she defaulted to the (mis)information in the chart: Patient is going to die.

It was by reading the records that I realized the "extra" nursing hours Bill had been able to get came from something called the Palliative Care Program. I finally understood why so many home care workers came with the notion that Bill was going to die. This service was provided with the very best of intentions, I believe, but it created endless extra miscommunication.

My list of discoveries went on. And on. And on.

A plethora of misinformation, miscommunication, and mistakes had plagued us through our entire journey. Though we accomplished an extraordinary life, under the circumstances, we could have avoided so many problems — medical, emotional, financial, and ultimately perhaps even Bill's death — had I known more about how to navigate the system from the outset.

The lessons I learned, often too late, about navigating the health care system could have saved us from much of the pain recounted in this story.

APPENDIX

PATIENT BEWARE

I DO NOT BELIEVE any professionals enter the health care realm to do harm. But harm happens. Often. According to the Health Canada Adverse Events Report, 2004, thousands of people die annually as a direct result of hospital mishaps. In 2004 the number was over 10,000. By 2006 that figure had risen dramatically, to 23,000. These figures are based solely on incident reports as filed only by hospital staff; many more incidents go unreported.

Thousands of those deaths were entirely preventable. I believe many of them happen, in part, because we, the public, do not know how to effectively advocate for ourselves.

Yes, our health care system is good. Excellent much of the time.

Yes, many thousands of dedicated, skilled, and noble professionals do their very best.

But it is a very imperfect system. Not omnipotent. Never infallible. We all need to be more cautious, more vigilant, and more involved in the management of our own care. Especially when we're in hospitals or long-term care facilities.

Anyone, and everyone, is at risk of being misdiagnosed, overmedicated, given an incorrect prognosis, and even of receiving inadequate follow-up care. Many people still believe they should simply do as they are told and should never question doctors. Often they simply don't know they have the right to ask about options and alternatives and the right to be very involved in the management of their own care. Patients who suffer cognitive issues, the elderly, and those who do not fit into a conventional diagnosis and treatment plan may be at even greater risk.

In this age of too few doctors, too little funding, and an aging population, knowing what to be watchful for, and how to effectively navigate the health care system, is essential. You absolutely must be, or have, your own advocate in order to attain optimum care and the best possible outcome.

Our story, as related in this book, became more complex than some, but it was by no means unique. Even in seemingly simple cases, things can go very, very wrong. Bill and I had always trusted the health care system. We could never have anticipated how badly it would fail us, or that I would have to battle this enormous, convoluted system for *his* life, *our* life, *our* future.

Looking back, and searching my husband's medical records, I realize many ways in which I could have protected him, and myself, from the mishaps, mistakes, and miscommunications we experienced. But the most important lesson is this all-important requirement of being or having an advocate. *What you don't know can hurt you.* Following are some of the lessons I learned, which I believe and hope will be valuable for others. They are written for the individual whose health is at stake but apply equally to all patients and their advocates.

Lesson #1: Be and stay healthy. This one of the most important things we can do. I believe that, because my husband was in great physical and emotional health, he was better prepared in 1992 to battle a serious illness and win. Be committed to good nutrition and exercise and avoid drug and alcohol abuse. Have regular health checkups. Learn to manage stress and problems in life. Be diligent about living a spiritually and emotionally well-balanced life. Enjoy life. It could save your life.

Lesson #2: Know your own medical information. Keep a written medical bio on hand and up to date. This is even more important than having a will and a power of attorney. It wastes time and leaves room for serious error when, in the midst of medical turmoil, details are given verbally, or forgotten. Give doctors as much information as possible: past illnesses, surgeries, family history, and, most importantly, the medications, supplements, and over-the-counter drugs you take and their dosage. Include your normal blood pressure, pulse, temperature, and respiration, because these numbers are different for everyone. Knowing, and communicating, your specific information is important. Make sure someone else knows where your medical information file is. Do this for children, too. You can't imagine how important this can be until you need it and don't have it.

Lesson #3: Follow the paperwork yourself, whether you are in a hospital, rehabilitation facility, or nursing home or are utilizing home care services. The domino effect of miscommunication is huge. In today's health care system, family doctors are rarely on staff in the hospital. They used to follow the details of your care. Now, *you* must be that cohesive link. Ask to go over your chart with a doctor or nurse daily. This is your opportunity to query any and all information, including tests and results, medications and changes, opinions and recommendations. Reports can go unread, be misinterpreted, or not be passed on to the right people. Ask to have consultation reports forwarded to you as well, and in a timely fashion. You need to be the most informed. You have the most at stake.

Lesson #4: Ask questions. You or your advocate must ask questions. Keep a journal; details get fuzzy quickly. Write out your questions for use in a medical facility or during a routine doctor's appointment. Knowing what to ask may require some homework, but it's worth it. Asking the right people is *vital*. Hospital residents and floor nurses may be very willing to answer, but it is safer, smarter, and likely more accurate to get your answers from the specialists and nurse managers. It is their responsibility to clarify information for you.

Lesson #5: Remember that prognosis is not an exact science. No one knows for sure what is possible. A prognosis is based on statistics and averages, experience and opinions. These factors can limit the options that are offered or recommended. Keep searching for therapies, activities, and other ideas that could improve progress and provide purpose and a better quality of life. Everyone's goal.

Lesson #6: Understand the basic 6 Ws of medications — Why, What, Who, When, With, and Without. Never accept medications without getting answers to these questions. In some cases you may choose to refuse on the basis of one or move of the 6 Ws. Talk to your primary physician or specialist, not their underlings, to voice your concerns and get your questions answered. This is the person who can change written orders. Never take medications without knowing what they are, and why they are prescribed.

Lesson #7: Gain access to the facility that best suits your needs. Patients, especially those living outside metropolitan areas, may not be given access to the specialists and specialties they need. Hospital policies can sometimes be followed at the expense of the patient. Do everything you can to insure you are in the facility that best suits your needs — with the appropriate staff, skills, and equipment. If you are somewhere unsuitable and meet only roadblocks, it may be necessary for you to call your Member of Parliament or the hospital CEO and even the media. It is the expertise that matters. *Do not* settle for less than you need, even if that means raising your voice. Scream and yell if you must.

Lesson #8: Follow your instincts. Listen to your gut when something or someone doesn't feel right. Well-meaning people can unwittingly create greater problems, so it is important for you to listen, learn, and question. Trust yourself, and follow up with the right people to resolve an issue. You won't always be right, but trusting yourself could very well help you avoid unnecessary pitfalls.

Lesson #9: Do not stay in a hospital or any other facility one hour more than is absolutely necessary. Going home as soon as possible can be a huge advantage for recovery: It can help you avoid hospital-transmitted infections and medication mishaps, as well as other potential problems related to a hospital stay. Older patients are at greater risk of being in bed for far too long, which can lead to muscle atrophy, cognitive issues, and pneumonia, one of the most common causes of death, which is often entirely avoidable if you get up and moving as soon as possible. While it is foolhardy to go home before it is safe, going home at the first legitimate opportunity is extremely important. Find out the treatment you would get staying in hospital and how much of that you could do, or get, at home. Home is usually safer, cleaner, and much better for sleeping. Even in extended-care centres, be watchful about medications and policies.

Lesson #10: Do your best to negotiate and convey your real needs. Medical professionals are just ordinary people doing their best in a very imperfect system. Money is often wasted on unimportant, even unnecessary, things, reducing the money available for staff and services. And much of the time and money that used to be spent on patient care is now spent on paperwork, much of this being the result of the lawsuit mentality we have developed. Because there is only so much money available, we all, including the administrators, must use these resources better in order to save lives, time, money, conflicts, and additional (avoidable) problems. We must demand more value and better care from our tax dollars.

Lesson #11: Educate yourself as much as possible and share your info with your primary physicians. This doesn't mean you should self-diagnose your problems — that can be very risky. But being involved with, and being taken seriously by, your medical team can require you to research your condition, question medications and adverse effects, and be informed about other possibilities. Find out what others have tried successfully. Never, ever stop looking for other options, other opinions, and other sources of hope.

Lesson #12: Invest in critical care insurance. It's as vital as death insurance, or more so. A policy that covers living expenses, extra care services, and rehabilitation services can save more than your bank account. Financial pressure when you are ill or injured makes everything more difficult. Coverage also often gives you a better choice of therapies and care. Be prepared.

Lesson #13: Practice good and open communication. Throughout a person's recovery from acute illness, an accident, or a lengthy illness, patients, supporting partners, and family can become tired, anxious, and overwhelmed. People can change under stress, and emotions can run high. Open dialogue between the patient (or advocate) and doctors, nurses, support people, and those in your inner circle can make an enormous difference. Don't be afraid to ask friends and professionals for help.

Lesson #14: Appoint your own advocate. Choose an advocate who will help you get what you need in health care, and who will fight for you in the event you are unable. Choose carefully, because being an advocate will require a commitment from them, and possibly the sharing of your medical information. It is also very helpful to have someone accompany you to medical appointments, because details and information can be overwhelming, confusing, and too difficult to remember. A second set of ears and eyes is invaluable. And never, ever go to the hospital alone.

CPSIA information can be obtained at www.ICGtesting.com
Printed in the USA
LVOW04s1226281114

415908LV00007B/18/P

9 781927 483961